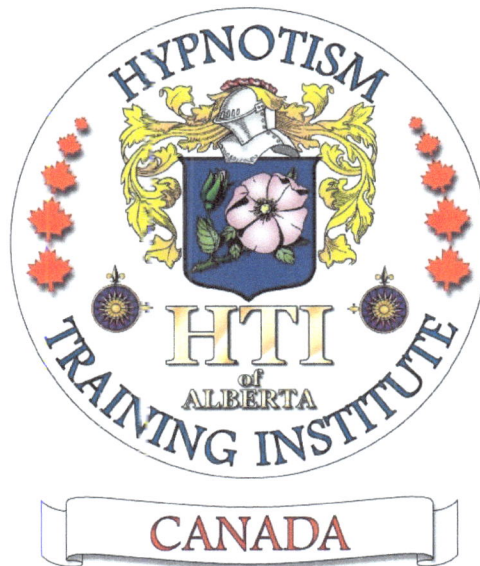

Hypnosis 601

Hypnotherapy And The Paranormal

By Anny J. Slegten

Hypnotherapy And The Paranormal
Anny Slegten
Published by
Kimberlite Publishing House
www.kimberlitePublishingHouse.com

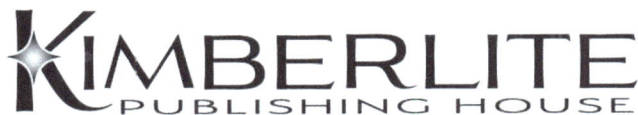

KIMBERLITE
PUBLISHING HOUSE

ISBN: 978-1-7752489-9-6

School Coat of Arms designed by Boomer Stralak
Book layout by Colin Christopher *www.colinchristopher.com*
Book cover and Kimberlite Logo designed by Marietta Miller
www.execugraphx.com

The Kimberlite-Diamond Connection

Kimberlite is a rock type that was first categorized over a 100 years ago based on descriptions of the diamond-bearing pipes of Kimberley, South Africa.

Kimberlites are the mechanism by which diamonds are brought to the surface.

Kimberlitic rocks are the most important primary source of diamonds and the main rock type in which significant diamond deposits have been found so far.

Anny is familiar with many rocks and minerals as her husband was raised around quarries, and later worked in several mines in Canada.

Therefore, it was natural for Anny to choose kimberlite as an analogy to the soul residing within our body – as a diamond within the kimberlite.

A Picture Is Worth A Thousand Words – The Amidah Buddha

The Amidah Buddha is venerated in Buddhist culture.

It represents unconditional love of self. Yes, you read it right: Unconditional love of self.

Although named differently in different countries and languages, you will have the same Buddha when asking for the Buddha representing unconditional love.

Deciding to take a new Reiki course, I went into a trance during the Reiki attunement. As I went into this deep trance - I asked Subby to let me know what was so important to have unconditional love of self.

The answer came to me crystal clear – and I was in shock! Unconditional love of self is a tall order, and has nothing to do with religion, or lack of it. Unconditional love is pertaining to the Paranormal.

This is the reason the Amidah Buddha was chosen for the cover of the book you hold in your hand right now: *Hypnotherapy and the Paranormal.*

In class, I will explain this to you in much greater detail.

With Love and Light,

Anny

Welcome to

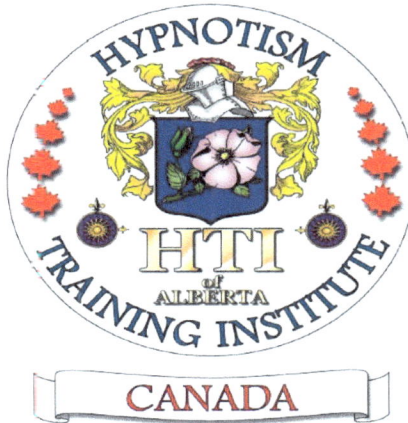

HYP 601 – Hypnotherapy And The Paranormal

This book belongs to:

Name _____

Mailing Address _____

_____

City or Town _____

Province/State _____ Postal Code/Zip _____

Country _____

Telephone   Home (___) _____   Work (___) _____

Instructor's Name: *Anny Slegten*

Today's Date: _____

Foreword

As you are taking this course, you are now entering the paranormal, and will discover a world alive and well – usually not seen with physical eyes.

Since Energy is everything and everything is Energy, you will be able to connect with everything possible, investigating events, and then heal whatever has to be healed – usually putting closures to various situations.

In this course, you will learn how to do:

- **Surrogate Sessions**
- **Consultation at a Distance, or 'Surrogate Consultation'**
- **Trance psychic ethical hypnotherapy at a distance**

When we are requested to investigate (and many times heal to) – these methods allow us to access information by connecting with the subjects' Universal Energy Field.

Being a Clinical Hypnotherapist in full time practice since 1984, I *"accidently"* initiated this therapeutic technique in 1986.

From simply investigating the reasons a business was not doing well, the session opened the complete Universe to a seldom understood reality: Energy is everything and everything is Energy.

That you believe or do not believe what I am teaching in this course is not the point.

The purpose is for you to understand and heal whatever situation the subject of the session finds itself into. This is for the clients' benefit, and you can bring closure to misunderstood situations, and many times – bring peace of mind.

As this subject is continuously updated, and to understand the various reasons clients are requesting surrogate sessions, please visit *www.success-and-more.com* and click on services.

Anny

Table Of Contents

A Note From Anny

Please remember:

The experiences derived from attending this course is a private and personal experience for each participant. As such please do respect the confidentiality of all participants and their remarks and actions and keep all such information private and confidential.

As a result, I am counting on you do your part at keeping this course environment safe and secure for all participants.

I am pleased to be able to supply transcripts of actual sessions. The intent and the information provided in this course are to enable you to help your client heal whatever comes up during a session. Remember, it is your client's session: Honour their truth.

The design and development of the Course Companion required the investment of substantial effort, time and money and is only intended for the participants of this course: HYP 601, Hypnotherapy and the Paranormal.

It is nice to see you here.

Enjoy!

Surrogate Session

The Facilitator

A surrogate session is teamwork. The better you work as a team, the more effective the session and the safer and enjoyable the working experience. **Remember: The facilitator's / hypnotherapist main purpose is to protect the surrogate.**

1. Be an observer.

   - Self
   - Surrogate
   - Client

2. Ask Surrogate: Anything about themselves they wish to transform and make better? Have it put into a container, close it, write on the side of the container what they want it to be transformed into, send it to the sun to be burned up, consumed and transformed into what they want, and know that by the time they leave your office, it will be done.

3. Lead the surrogate into a hypnotic trance.

4. Ask for protection and affirm the surrogate's space, as well as what they want for themselves, and proceed accordingly.

5. Ask the surrogate to check the "security" of their own aura as well as the facilitator's, the room they are in, the office building, the property, below the building as well as above the building.

6. Ask the surrogate to bring the client in front of them.

7. Ask the surrogate: "Anything required to keep the client's energy separated or contained"?

Your Notes

Anny's Teaching

8. Ask the surrogate: "Anything required to keep the client's energy separated or contained"?

9. Begin the session.

10. Ask surrogate "What do you see or what is coming to your awareness" and proceed as for a "regular" hypnotherapy session. Remember to stay an observer, remind the surrogate they are reporting the client's conditions, experiences and feelings, and keep an eye on client's picture.

11. Prior to wrap it up, ask "anything else" or if client has a wish, what would it be?

12. Wrap up the session and release the subject you worked on back to their own space.

13. Allow surrogate to say anything else they would like about the session. Remember, it is the client's session. Be considerate and keep any predictions between the surrogate and yourself after shutting off the recording.

14. Shut off the recording. And wrap it up with the surrogate.

15. Deepen the trance. Remember, the facilitator's main purpose is to protect the surrogate. Do whatever is required for the well-being of the surrogate. Do this quickly.

16. Ask the surrogate to check their own aura, your own aura, the room you are occupying, inside, under and above the office building office, as well as the property.

17. Ask the surrogate "Anything else"?

18. Thank the universe and guide the surrogate out of the trance.

Your Notes

Anny's Teaching

Surrogate Session

The Surrogate

A surrogate session is team work. The better you work as a team, the more effective the session and the safer and enjoyable the working experience. **Remember: The surrogate's/reporter's purpose is to report what is seen, felt and smelled to the facilitator. Trust what comes. Report things as is and stay an observer.**

Following the facilitator recommendation, first dispose or transform whatever you wish.

1. Be an observer and secure in your own space.

2. Remember at all times it is the client's session, and "stay out of it".

3. Check your feelings about doing the session.

4. Enjoy the experience of being let into a hypnotic trance.

5. Ask for protection and affirm your space.

6. Bring the subject you will work with in front of you.

7. Secure your own space.

8. Trust what comes and "stay out of it". Report **as is** what you see, feel and smell. Remember, it is the subject's session.

9. This session is recorded. Therefore, report the session as it unfolds.

Your Notes

Anny's Teaching

10. Put the subject you worked on back together.

11. Release client into their own space

12. Report whatever you fell is appropriate. Remember, it is the client's session: Be considerate and only share your predictions of the outcome of the session with the facilitator after the recording has been shut off.

13. Be aware of your feelings and be honest with yourself.

14. The facilitator's main purpose is to protect the surrogate. Ask whatever you feel is required for your well-being and allow the facilitator to do so quickly.

15. Trust your intuition and do whatever you feel is appropriate for the facilitator and for yourself

16. Enjoy the satisfaction of a job well done.

Please note:
This therapeutic technique requires two hypnotherapists trained in this modality.

Sometimes, there is no-one available where you are. Therefore, a person you know goes into a deep trance and stays objective may be the surrogate.

When hiring a person not trained in this modality, **<u>it is important that you are the facilitator</u>**

As well, to keep clarity of thoughts, perform a maximum of two surrogate sessions a day as a surrogate or a facilitator.

Your Notes

Anny's Teaching

© Hypnotism Training Institute of Alberta

Does Consciousness Exist Outside Of The Brain?

In my books The Four Mental Agreements to Losing Weight, as well as Stories from the Other Side, Conversations with Those who Passed Away, I wrote about the brain and the mind, and by now, you must have noticed that I keep talking about the mind, that non-physical part of us.

Have you ever thought how come we can see something in our mind and it manifests?

A Canadian, Dr Penfield was the founder of the Montreal Neurological Institute and one of the greatest neuroscientists who ever lived. After years of research, Dr. Penfield discovered and confirmed the mind is not physical and has a different function than the brain, that physical part of us.

Yes, we are more than flesh and bones.

The mind, our thoughts are non-physical and the brain is physical.

Therefore, the mind needs a fully functional brain to successfully "download" an information, a command to our awareness.

The command is a perception you can describe; a picture the mind sends to the brain.

Although physical, the function of the brain is truly magical.

Your Notes

Anny's Teaching

For example, below is an excellent article explaining this by Clifford N. Lazarus PHD on Psychology Today:

Original Source Materials:

https://www.psychologytoday.com/ca/blog/think-well/201906/does-consciousness-exist-outside-the-brain

Is consciousness actually a property of the universe like gravity or light?

The prevailing consensus in neuroscience is that consciousness is an emergent property of the brain and its metabolism. When the brain dies, the mind and consciousness of the being to whom that brain belonged ceases to exist. In other words, without a brain there can be no consciousness.

But according to the decades-long research of Dr. Peter Fenwick, a highly regarded neuropsychiatrist who has been studying the human brain, consciousness, and the phenomenon of near death experience (NDE) for 50 years, this view is incorrect. Despite initially being highly incredulous of NDEs and related phenomena, Fenwick now believes his extensive research suggests that consciousness persists after death. In fact, Fenwick believes that consciousness actually exists independently and outside of the brain as an inherent property of the universe itself like dark matter and dark energy or gravity.

Hence, in Fenwick's view, the brain does not create or produce consciousness; rather, it filters it. As odd as this idea might seem at first, there are some analogies that bring the concept into sharper focus. For example, the eye filters and interprets only a very small sliver of the electromagnetic spectrum and the ear registers only a narrow range of sonic frequencies. Similarly, according to Fenwick, the brain filters and perceives only a tiny part of the cosmos' intrinsic "consciousness."

Indeed, the eye can see only the wavelengths of electromagnetic energy that correspond to visible light. But the entire EM spectrum is vast and extends from extremely low energy, long wavelength radio waves to incredibly energetic, ultrashort-wavelength gamma rays. So, while we can't actually "see" much of the EM spectrum, we know things like X-rays, infrared radiation, and microwaves exists because we have instruments for detecting them.

Similarly, our ears can register only a narrow range of sonic frequencies but we know a huge amount of others imperceptible to the human ear exist nevertheless.

When the eye dies, the electromagnetic spectrum does not vanish or cease to be; it's just that the eye is no longer viable and therefore can no longer filter, be stimulated by, and react to light energy. But the energy it previously interacted with remains nonetheless. And so too when the ear dies, or stops transducing sound waves, the energies that the living ear normally respond to still exist. According to Fenwick, so it is with consciousness. Just because the organ that filters, perceives, and interprets it dies does not mean the phenomenon itself ceases to exist. It only ceases to be in the now-dead brain but continues to exist independently of the brain as an external property of the universe itself.

What is more, according to Fenwick, our consciousness tricks us into perceiving a false duality of self and other when in fact there is only unity. We are not separate from other aspects of the universe but an integral and inextricable part of them. And when we die, we transcend the human experience of consciousness, and its illusion of duality, and merge with the universe's entire and unified property of consciousness. So, ironically, only in death can we be fully conscious.

This is not to be taken as joining God or a creator because the cosmic 1consciousness that Fenwick describes did not create the universe but is simply a property of it. Obviously, despite his impressive body of research into this subject, there is no current way to empirically establish the validity of Fenwick's cosmic consciousness hypothesis. Ultimately, it aligns more with faith than science.

Your Notes

Thus it seems the answer to the question in this post's title is "No." There is no empirically established explanatory framework for understanding how consciousness can exist independently and outside of the brain.

Recall the old riddle, "If a tree falls in the woods and no one is there to hear it, does it still make a sound?" Well, it seems the answer is "No." Because sound is the conscious perception of sonic or acoustic stimuli that requires a sense organ to experience. Without an ear to hear and a brain to interpret the stimulation there will be only molecular vibrations but no sound, per se. In the same vein, all of the energies and biophysical phenomena that the brain experiences as consciousness do indeed exist independently and outside of the brain (e.g., physics, chemistry and quantum events). But the wondrous experience of consciousness itself seems to require a brain to give rise to it and a brain-based mind to perceive it.

Remember: Think well; Act well; Feel well; Be well!

Your Notes

Anny's Teaching

More Inductions – Remote Viewing

Three induction techniques as performed during Remote Viewing courses.

I genuinely enjoyed the in-person courses in Remote Viewing by David Morehouse.

What was most interesting to me was the inductions that were narrated to get us in and hypnotic trance, the reason I am sharing them with you.

I was obvious these inductions were aimed at getting the most reluctant attendants to go into an altered state of awareness, although for the four hypnotherapists attending the course, it made us every time go into quite a ride!

We will begin with a short breath training exercise.

During this exercise you will be asked to breathe in a controlled and deliberate manner.

First, as you inhale, loosen the muscles at the back of your throat and your nasal passages. Breathe slowly through your nose, as though you were smelling a beautiful flower and then exhale softly through your nose.

Keep your mouth and jaw relaxed to the point that your front teeth do not touch. Gently press your lips together. Do not tighten them or press them together.

Breath in such a relaxed manner that the air you inhale strikes the back of the throat first, creating a sensation that it never passed through the nose at all.

As you breath in, your body should rhythmically move in such a way that your belly will rise first, then your rib cage and finally your upper chest.

Concentrate on this as you breathe. Your belly rises, then your ribs and then your upper chest.

Now release, slowly exhaling through your nose again. Take a few moments to practice this on your own. Inhale slowly, a complete breath and then release. Continue on your own for a moment and then I'll rejoin you.

(Pause)

We are now going to use our breath to cleanse as we meditate.

Listen to the sound of my voice, rest quietly and for the next few minutes continue paying very close attention to your breathing.

For now, think of nothing else but your breathing. At first, your mind may have a tendency to wander. Let it do so.

But gently bring your awareness back to your breathing. Always to your breathing and hold your attention there. Listen to the rhythm of your breathing. Be aware of it. Be aware that as you listen each breath will lengthen.
Your rhythm grows slower as your body softens and begins to allowing each breath to flow easily through your cycle.

As you inhale, continue doing it through your nose, only this time pause briefly, holding your breath as it cleanses.

Now release it through your mouth as though you were gently blowing out a candle. Inhale through your nose. Hold it until I say release. Then exhale through your mouth.

Ready – inhale, breathe deeply. Watch the breath come into your body, gradually filling your lungs with the life force of the universe.

Your Notes

Anny's Teaching

Hold the breath, now release, exhale through your mouth, releasing all your tensions and anxieties, releasing all the negative thoughts and energy with your breath.

Inhale, watch your breath once again. Let the universal energy of spirit fill your lungs. Hold it for a moment.

Now release. Releasing with the breath al your tensions and worries.

Breathe in slowly and with your mind's eye, carefully watch as the breath gradually fills your lungs, hold the breath again, be thankful for it.

Now release and cleanse your body of all negative energies, thoughts and the worries as you exhale.

Again, breathe in slowly and deeply through your nose, hold your breath, be thankful for it and now release it, expelling any thoughts or worries that may impact on your clarity of thoughts. Cleanse yourself with your breath in this phase of life.

Breathe in the gift of life. Accept it as it energizes every cell of your body. Hold the breath and now release, expelling from your body anything which might cause you to worry or to think negatively about any one or anything. Slowly and deliberately breathe in again and be reminded that the essence of your being is the practice of gratitude.

Recognize that you are alive only to the degree that you are moved by the title rhythm of receiving and giving.

Release your gossamer curtain, the veil hanging in a window separating time and eternity, blowing back and forth in an endless dance of breath.

Continue this breathing exercise at your own rhythm for a while as you surrender to the movement of your breath and your body.

Your mind will begin to change. It will clear and where you once were acting, you will soon be moved by a power beyond yourself.

Your Notes

Anny's Teaching

The rhythm of your breath tells you that you are of the same substance as the spirit that moves everything within the matrix of all creation. Practice on your own for a while and I will rejoin you in a moment.

We will now begin a short yoga relaxation exercise.

Scan your body beginning with your head, your scalp, from your forehead from the top of your head to the base of the back of your neck.

Relax all of the muscles covering your head. Relax them all. No tension is present at all. Relax them. Let them go loose.

Now move to the area around your ears and focus there. Relaxing the muscles around your ears, letting go of any tension that you find there. All of the mini muscles surrounding your ears, let them relax. Let them go.

Now focus on the area around your eyes and the muscles surrounding the eyes and nose. Relax them. Let them unwind, letting go of any tension you might find there. As you progress through this exercise, continue your breathing as you have been instructed.

Now focus on the muscles around your mouth, jaw and lips. Let go of any tension found there. Imagine the muscles unwinding as a coil of rubber bands would let go of any tension or pressure. Relax the muscles in your tongue and down your throat into your esophagus, releasing any tension or pressure you might find there.

Follow your next breath through your esophagus and into your stomach. As you exhale, release any tension or pressure you find. Do this three more times on your own and I will rejoin you.

(pause)

Your Notes

Anny's Teaching

Now bring your awareness back to the outside of your body, to your neck and search for any tension or tightness in the muscles and nerves and vessels of your neck. Be aware of any sensations and let go of any tension you find there. Cleansing and purging it from your body as you exhale.

Now bring your focus, your awareness on your chest and all the thousands of muscles and nerves and vessels that wrap themselves around your body at this point.
As you exhale, release any tension you may find there.

Now shift your awareness to your back. To the area across your shoulders. To the joints of your shoulders and of your upper arms. Scan this area and release any tension as you breathe. Release any tension or tightness you may find there. Be aware of this area and all of its sensations.

Continue to bring your awareness down your arms to your forearms and elbows, releasing and cleansing as you slowly scan this part of your body. Breath in and breath out, cleansing away any tension or pressure. Continue to shift your awareness downward into your hands and your forearms and your wrists, sensing any pressure or soreness found in the mini joints, nerves and muscles of your hands. Breathe deeply, slowly and release, expelling any tension or pressure you may find in your hands.

Bring your awareness to your spinal cord and slowly trace your spine. Relax each of the muscles surrounding each vertebrae. Trace the spine in your mind's eye from the base of your skull to the tip of your tailbone. Scanning for any tension or pressure or sensation. If you find any sore places or tight spots, spend a moment to focus on them and cleanse them with your breathing. Rid yourself of any tension found there. Do this and I will rejoin you shortly.

(pause)

Your Notes

Anny's Teaching

Now focus your attention to your hips and groin area. Release any tension found there as you breath.

Now move your awareness to the large muscles of your buttocks. Relax these muscles and release any tension you might find there. Be aware of the subtle changes you feel.

Now bring your awareness to the muscles and those of your thighs, scanning down the thighs towards your knees, releasing any tension or pressure.

As you do this, continue to concentrate on your breathing, cleansing your body's tension anywhere you might find it.

If you fall asleep, it is okay because you will still hear my voice and your body will still react.

Move into the area of your knees, being sensitive to the many nerves, muscles and blood vessels surrounding these joints. Scan them carefully, releasing any tension, soreness or pressure found there. Heal this. Breathe in and release anything negative with your breath.

Now slowly shift your awareness down to your calves. Searching for and releasing any tension found there. Move into your ankles and feet, scanning the mini muscles and nerves found there. If you find any tension, focus on it, release it, and expel it from your body with your breath.

Now scan one last time all the muscles of your body for any tension or pressure. If you find any, again, focus on it, release it and let go of it, cleansing it with your breath.

(pause)

Your Notes

Anny's Teaching

Now shift your awareness to your internal organs, to your heart and lungs. Scan here for any tightness or pressure and relax this area as you breathe. Let the muscles relax, letting go of every pressure, no matter how slight.

Now shift your awareness to your intestines, your liver, your spleen and all the vital organs found there in your abdomen. Scan them, releasing any tension or pressure found there.

Breathe deeply, cleansing and relaxing these parts of your body.

Now feel your skin. Be aware of your body's largest organ and all of the sensations present there. Scan your entire body, softly searching for any pressure or tension. Become aware of it and then cleanse it from your body as you breathe. Very well. You are now in a state of complete and total relaxation.

Your Notes

Anny's Teaching

The Kundalini

The following is an explanation retrieved from the web:

The Kundalini is imagined as a coiled serpent lying asleep at the base of our spine. Kundalini is the dormant energy within us that expands our awareness. Kundalini is regarded as the greatness of which we are each capable.

We become aware of our creative capacities and our radiant caliber. We become aware of our finite relationship with infinity. Kundalini makes it possible for us as humans with finite identities to relate to our infinite identities.

When the glandular system is activated and the nervous system is strong the energies of the two systems combine to create a movement or flow in the spinal fluid, a sensitivity in the nerve endings. The "brain in its totality receives signals and integrates them." Kundalini yoga is an ancient technology designed to expand our awareness. Our capacities and choices are determined by our awareness.

As we expand our awareness, we are able to go beyond our perceived conscious limits; we are empowered to make more daring choices; we have the energy to create bountiful and exciting lives.

From what I have observed in my years of practice, the Kundalini opens up and expands naturally as we evolve. It does it safely and at its own pace.

Major emotional and mental problems develop when one does physical and breathing exercises to force the Kundalini to open up before the emotional and nervous system is ready for it. It is like taking the moth out of the cocoon.

The result is mentally devastating.

Your Notes

Anny's Teaching

The Tree Of Life Talking Boards (Ouija)

The Ouija board is a form of communication having been used for centuries by some of the U.K.s best pioneer mediums of past years, but has grown a reputation for being a tool never to be used, with an unjustified attachment of mysticism. This is not the case according to the psychics who use regularly the Ouija board.

These tree of life (Ouija) boards have become the chosen tool of thousands in and around the U.K proving that some of the oldest methods are still the most reliable to prove life after death.

You may use the Ouija board anytime you feel the urge to do so either with a group of friends, a family get together or a personal time for you alone. It is usually performed at night and starts with respectfully requesting an Energy, a Spirit to come to "work" the Ouija board and give the information and/or guidance to your question.

As the Ouija board comes to life, you are realizing that you are having a séance with the energy of a spirit who has decided to answer your call.

Your Notes

Anny's Teaching

Clients Who Say: "I Do Not Know"

There are many ways to help a client when, no matter what you do, a client will answer "I do not know", usually avoiding feeling.

1. Ask the client to describe the issue they would like to have healed.

2. Ask them: "Where does it sit in their body".

This is often easy as the client will feel tension or pain in an area of the body whenever they think about the issue.

Ask them to describe the feeling, shape, color, texture, OR weight.

Does it make a sound?

Without realizing it, this usually gets the client out into their feelings.

Your Notes

Anny's Teaching

Pecans In The Cemetery

On the outskirts of a small town, there was a big, old pecan tree just inside the cemetery fence. One day, two boys filled up a bucketful of nuts and sat down by the tree, out of sight, and began dividing the nuts.

'One for you, one for me, one for you, one for me,' said one boy. Several dropped and rolled down toward the fence.

Another boy came riding along the road on his bicycle. As he passed, he thought he heard voices from inside the cemetery. He slowed down to investigate. Sure enough, he heard, *'One for you, one for me, one for you, one for me...'*

He just knew what it was. He jumped back on his bike and rode off. Just around the bend he met an old man with a cane, hobbling along.

'Come here quick,' said the boy, *'you won't believe what I heard! Satan and the Lord are down at the cemetery dividing up the souls!'*

The man said, *'Beat it kid, cannot you see it is hard for me to walk'* When the boy insisted though, the man hobbled slowly to the cemetery.

Standing by the fence they heard, *'One for you, one for me. One for you, one for me.'*

The old man whispered, *'Boy, you have been telling me the truth. Let us see if we can see the Lord...?'*

www.success-and-more.com

Shaking with fear, they peered through the fence, yet were still unable to see anything. The old man and the boy gripped the wrought iron bars of the fence tighter and tighter as they tried to get a glimpse of the Lord.

At last they heard, *'One for you, one for me. That is all. Now let us go get those nuts by the fence and we will be done...'*

They say the old man had the lead for a good half-mile before the kid on the bike passed him.

E-mail received from Attila May 23, 2012

Your Notes

Anny's Teaching

Imagine This Happening

A lesson to be learned from one typing the wrong email address!

A Minneapolis couple decided to go to Florida to thaw out during a particularly icy winter. They planned to stay at the same hotel where they spent their honeymoon 20 years earlier. Because of hectic schedules, it was difficult to coordinate their travel schedules.

So, the husband left Minnesota and flew to Florida on Thursday, with his wife flying down the following day.

The husband checked into the hotel. There was a computer in his room, so he decided to send an email to his wife. However, he accidentally left out one letter in her email address, and without realizing his error, sent the email.

Meanwhile, somewhere in Houston, a widow had just returned home from her husband's funeral. He was a minister who was called home to glory following a heart attack.

The widow decided to check her email expecting messages from relatives and friends. After reading the first message, she screamed and fainted. The widow's son rushed into the room, found his mother on the floor, and saw the computer screen which read:

Your Notes

To: My Loving Wife

Subject: I have Arrived Date: October 16, 2004

I know you are surprised to hear from me. They have computers here now and you are allowed to send emails to your loved ones. I have just arrived and have been checked in. I see that everything has been prepared for your arrival tomorrow. Looking forward to seeing you then! Hope your journey is as uneventful as mine was.

P.S. Sure is freaking hot down here!

Jamie Bryant
YR Radio Creative/Swing
jbryant@ab.ncc.ca
ph: (780) 723-4461
fax: (780) 723-3765

Your Notes

Anny's Teaching

Ramtha On Remote Viewing And Knowing The Future

Excerpts from Ramtha newsletter received April 2, 2009

"When students were learning how to do sending-and-receiving, the sending partner created an image in the frontal lobe. As the sending partner created the image, the receiving partner focused on their partner's face and held their face in their frontal lobe. As they held their face in the frontal lobe, what their partner was doing was brought to the attention of the midbrain and behind their face appeared an image. They drew the image and look how many of them got it correct. It is called reading someone else's mind. Are you impressed?

"Would you be impressed if I told you that the sending partner could create the most difficult mathematical equation and it did not matter if the receiving partner knew math at all? All they would have to do is focus on their partner's face and know the answer. And they do it. You should be impressed, because what happens when you develop this faculty? What can you not know?"

– Ramtha
May 1997

Excerpts from: Ramtha, *In the Beginning*. Ramtha's School of Enlightenment. May 3-4, 1997. Copyright © 1997 JZ Knight,

Your Notes

Anny's Teaching

"The reason we get information ahead of time is because we have a pause in the frontal lobe, which means that the computer program isn't running continuously in the neocortex. Someone has pushed the pause button on the neocortex. That causes a blank screen to appear in the frontal lobe. As soon as we have a blank screen, the brain automatically moves to the next level, which is always the midbrain. Then you will get a flash. In a moment you will see something. You will see it not with these eyes but see it with the brain. Remember, I told you that it is not the eyes that see; it is the brain that sees."

"Psychic people are psychic because they have developed an ability from early childhood to be still and quiet. A trance state is a self-willed state. The trance state means stilling or paralyzing the sensory perception in the neocortex. When you do, the next level opens up in the brain and you start to get information. How many of you understand? So be it. And is it possible to change precognitive experiences? Yes, it is."

– Ramtha
August 1996

Excerpt from: Ramtha, *The Mystical Brain*. Ramtha's School of Enlightenment. August 13, 1996. Copyright © 1996 JZ Knight

Your Notes

Anny's Teaching

Anny's Special And Relaxing Induction

First, make sure it is safe for you to close your eyes while listening to this self hypnosis recording.

Please make yourself as comfortable as possible, loosen clothes that bind you. Now that you are comfortable, listen to the sound of my voice. Follow my instructions, and you will have the most enjoyable experience. Please note that your subconscious mind will be receptive to the suggestions you are hearing, even if you seem to fall asleep while listening to the sound of my voice.

Now stare at a point on the ceiling overhead. Stare at a point on the ceiling overhead. Take a deep breathe. Exhale ..., take another deep breathe ..., exhale ... .

And as you take another deep breathe ..., and exhale ..., close your eyes ..., you will keep your eyes closes until I ask you to open them.

Now I am asking for your protection and wellbeing, and I say "Got, please allow only good things to come to us. And for this blessing, we give thanks".

And now, become aware of your light. The light of yours, it is like a mini sun in your chest. Some people can see it, some people can feel it, some people simply know it is there.

That light of yours, that mini sun in your chest. Let it shine, let it shine, let it shine throughout every part of your body, throughout your aura, cleansing your body, cleansing your aura, strengthening your body, strengthening your aura, extending itself at one arm length in front of you, behind you, above you, beneath you, and at each side of you and mentally repeat with me, claiming dominion over your space:

"This is my body, this is my space, only light can come to me, only light can come from me, only my light can be here".

Take a deep breathe ..., exhale ..., sleep now.
Inhale ..., exhale ..., sleep now.

When I say, "Sleep now", this is not the sleep you experience when you fall asleep. I am talking about a hypnotic sleep when your subconscious mind is open and receptive to the suggestions you are receiving.

As you take another deep breath, and exhale, you become aware of a staircase, a beautiful staircase, a very beautiful staircase ..., you stand at the top of the stairs and you notice how it looks as you look from the top down. In your mind place your hand on the railing and you notice how it feels in the palm of your hand.

Slowly you begin to walk down the stairs ..., one step at a time. One step at a time, and with each step you take, you tell yourself that you are becoming more and more relaxed, and with each step you take, you become more and more comfortable. When at the bottom of the staircase, standing on the last step, in your mind, turn around and as you look up notice how different the staircase looks from the bottom than it did from the top. And you realize: This is what life is all about. It is the way we perceive things that makes our reality.

In your mind, as you turn and step off the last step you become aware of a chalkboard with all different colours of chalk. You walk toward the board and pick up the right colour of chalk for you. You begin to write the numbers from 10 down to the number one. With each number that you write on the board, you go deeper and deeper into relaxation. With each number you write you become more and more relaxed. And when you are finished writing the number one, you set the piece of chalk down and pick up the eraser.

You begin at the number 10, and erase the number off the board, slowly erasing the numbers down to number one. With each number that you erase, you become more and more relaxed. With each number your erase

Your Notes

Anny's Teaching

you tell yourself that you become more and more comfortable, more and more relaxed.

When you are finished erasing the last number, you become aware of a doorway. You walk towards the doorway, and you notice how the frame of the door looks, the colour of the door, and as you get near the door you tell yourself that on the other side of this door is the place that suggests total and complete relaxation to you. You know that this doorway will lead you to a place that is perfect for you, where you are completely safe and totally, totally at peace within yourself and the world around you.

In your mind, as you stand in front of the door, you notice how the door handle feels in your hand, you turn the handle to open the door before you, and you notice how the door sounds as you close the door behind you.

You walk into the perfect place, that suggests complete and total relaxation for you. Total and complete relaxation. And just be there. Be there and enjoy that feeling that is becoming so familiar to you, so familiar …, so relaxing …, and you feel wonderfully good.

As you are there, notice how you feel..., how comfortable you are, how relaxed you have become. This place is just for you, with everything that you have ever hoped for. In this place you are exactly the person you want to be, in your mind you are comfortable, and you are safe. Just be there. Just be there.

During this session the sound of my voice will make you go deeper and deeper into relaxation, deeper and deeper..., and the familiar sounds of the room will make you go deeper and deeper into relaxation. Just enjoy that familiar feeling of relaxation that is becoming so familiar to you.

Just enjoy this special place, this place that is completely yours to go to whenever you want to feel at peace with yourself and with the world around you, feeling comfortable and so relaxed. Safe and just enjoying this space that suggests complete relaxation to you.

As your subconscious mind is open and receptive to the suggestions that you are receiving now, is sorting all things out and is making all the necessary improvements right now that you desire and improving your life in a most delightful and positive way.

Be there. Feel it.

And when it is safe for you to close your eyes and fall asleep, remember how relaxed and comfortable you feel right now.

Simply remember the sound of my voice, and as you take a slow deep breathe, and exhale, close your eyes and fall into the most wonderful sleep.

As your subconscious mind is sorting all things out, and will improve whatever it feels can be improved, allowing your body and emotions to be calm, cool, and relaxed. So that you can live fully, physically, emotionally, mentally, spiritually, and financially.

That is right!

And watch the magic fall out of the sky with pleasure, joy, comfort, ease, grace and gratitude, your hearth full of love.

To wake up on time, feeling refreshed, relaxed, renewed, totally at peace with yourself, and with the world around you. And so it is. And so it is.

And now I am going to count from one to five and then I will say, your eyes are open, you are fully aware. Very refreshed, relaxed, renewed, enjoying a sharp mind, healthy body, tranquil heart, and a clear head.

One, slowly calmly gently easily you begin to return to full awareness once again. Enjoying a sharp mind, clear head, and tranquil heart.

Two, each muscle and nerve in your body is loose, limp, and relaxed and you feel wonderfully good. You feel at peace with yourself, and with the world around you, enjoying a sharp mind, clear head, and a tranquil heart.

Your Notes

Anny's Teaching

Three, from head to toe, you are feeling much better in every way. Physically better, mentally better, emotionally cool, calm, and serene. Enjoying a sharp mind, clear head, and tranquil heart.

Four your eyes begin to feel sparkling clean, as if they were bathed in cool spring water.

And five. Eyes open..., open your eyes.

You are fully aware. Take a slow deep breathe. Fill up your lungs and stretch!!

www.success-and-more.com

Your Notes

Anny's Teaching

Questions About Chris's Session

- Question 1 -

- Question 2 -

- Question 3 -

- Question 4 -

- Question 5 -

Transcript – Surrogate Session for Chris

Concern: un unhealthy attitude

Although in his 30's, Chris is like 2 people:
- A regular, responsible man then changes personality
and becomes a teenager as soon as one of "the boys" calls him.

Facilitator: It is November 19th in the year 2004.
This is a healing at a distance session for Chris at the request of his girlfriend and the time is now 9:07 PM.

And this is a session that is meant to be healing session for everyone concerned.

And are you ready?

Anny: Okay. All right.

Lead the surrogate into a trance.

Facilitator: Take a deep breath and close your eyes.

And as you close your eyes, you feel your body sinking deeper into the chair, relaxing all the muscles, the nerves, the bones in your body. As you feel that wonderful state of hypnosis flowing over your body, relaxing your mind.

Asking for protection and affirm the surrogate's space

And I am asking for your protection and well being and I say, God, please allow only to come to us. And for this blessing, we give thanks and now you ask to be put into the protection of your light. Your very own spark of life. At the centre of your chest. Let it shine, let it shine. Let it shine throughout every cell of your body. Throughout your aura. Cleansing your body, cleansing your aura. Strengthening your body, strengthening your aura. And extending itself at one arm's length above you, beneath you, at each side of you, in front of you and behind you. And mentally repeat with me, this is my body, this is my space, only light can come to me. Only light can come from me. This is my body and this is my space. Only my light is here.

Ask the surrogate to check the "security" of their own aura.

And now please check your aura and mine as well to make sure it is good for this type of work.

Anny: Your aura is quite nice and mine is good too.

And I must say, Chris is here.

Facilitator: Okay.

Anny: He is looking at me with huge eyes. Yah, he is here.

Get permission from client's higher self to proceed with the session.

Facilitator: I would like you to ask him for his permission to do this healing session and as a healing session for him, to heal him physically, mentally, emotionally and spiritually.

Anny: Yes, he is like…

Oh yah, he knows what is going on here. He knows what is the purpose of the whole thing and he is scared. There is scare in his eyes. A feel in his eyes I should say. Yah, he is…

Facilitator:: So what is going on? What is he scared of?

Anny: All right, it is because for him. I am going all the way back to the decision to be popular.

It is very important to be popular and I see him – he went straight back as a young boy and then... .

He is a young boy, then a teenager.

Extremely popular to be, important to be popular. Very important. Popular with his friends. So, the thing is, it is something about Chris. He likes to be liked. To be approved of by his friends.

The thing is that …, just a moment Chris, I am going to show you something here.
Let us say you observe someone who is doing very well and you see the supposed friends from far away.

You know when you distance yourself, you can tell what they are doing.

They are destroying somebody because they do not want that person to improve. And what would you tell that person?

You know what? he knows.

He says, I know, I know.

He says, yah, I know. The thing is there is also a fear to get older. There is also a fear to get older because…

Facilitator: So what does that mean to him?

Anny: What?

Facilitator: Getting older – what does that mean?

Anny: Well, it is because getting older – for whatever reason, getting older is no fun.

Well, where did you get that?

Well, he shows me the commercials that he was watching when he was a teenager.

The guys around the campfire, drinking and laughing and singing and you know – you could call it horsing around, you know. Guy together doing that. Doing guy things. The thing is, Chris that is a commercial to make you buy beer.

Facilitator: Umm hum.

Anny: That is all.

Facilitator: Can you see…. Can you have him look at his life and see how the belief, the need, the feeling is very important to be popular or that fear of his getting older because there is no fun and how has that affected decisions that he has made in his life? And how is that affecting his life today?

Anny: All right.
He is…, huh – is not that interesting.

He says that is how come he will not cut ties and he shows me a girl. He said it is because you know he is very fearful. He is fearful of moving ahead so to speak, but it is in age. It is not anything. There is something in age here. He... for him, there is something about staying young with staying popular with your gang so to speak.

So he is showing me a few things there.

I say yah, but you know what. Have a look at what they do. Those people are no friend to you. They are no friends to you.

So now I am going to put Chris on stage so to speak. All by himself there. So I can have a good look at him... And you know what, that Chris is quite fearful.

Facilitator:: Umm hum.

Anny: There is a fear there... Ohh

Facilitator: Where does that fear come from? I would like for him to go back. All the way back to the beginning of the fear.

Anny: He has been given away.

Facilitator: Umm.

Anny: And you know Chris, sometimes in life, for whatever reason, because your mother gave you away is one thing. The thing is that... what was going on in her life. What was going on in her life so that she had to give you away? And that is the thing. It has nothing to do with you Chris, it has something to do with what was going on in her life.

Facilitator: And perhaps after he sees that, we do always choose our parents when we come down. Perhaps he can go a little further back to before he came to start this life and see why he chose a mother that would give him away. Maybe he can look and see what the purpose of all of that was.

Anny: Okay, I am back into the planning stage here. And there is something about Chris' disposition. The disposition of his soul. It is not being able to say no.

Facilitator: Umm, umm hum.

Anny: You know what Chris, not being true to yourself. That is what it is, you are not true to yourself.

So now Chris, have a look at you, at your essence and have a look at all those supposed friends and I am going to ask you to go into their heads, okay because there are friends there and they are, they all have a rope around Chris because they want to drown him, so to speak.

So, I am going to ask Chris here. Here is Chris here. I say, okay Chris take a deep breath and as you exhale, go into that one's head. There is one with an angular face there.

Facilitator: Umm hum.

Anny: Okay. I will ask him to go into his head and look at his intent as he is roping you like that. Look at his intent. Have a good look as you are looking at that guy's head. Uhh huhh.

Facilitator: And what is he seeing?

Anny: He is very jealous. Extremely jealous and will do everything so that he loses his job and he loses his girlfriend. Umm hum. He will do everything.

So take a deep breath and get out of there. Chris. He is shaking his head, like that – oohhh…

So take a deep breath now and let us go into the other one's head. Okay, that one has – the one that I see now has quite a wide forehead, but the jaw – the thing goes a little bit like that, but the other one was not like that. But this one has a higher forehead. A wider forehead so to speak. Here, but like this (gesturing a short and pointed chin) Whatever. Okay, and he goes into his head now and look at what is going on.

You know what, Chris is very scared of what he is finding out in there, let me tell you, because I can feel his – ohhhh..,. okay, umm hum…

Get out of there.

Now it feels better when out of there, uhh huhh…
And now there is another one. Okay, from what I am getting. The third one he is looking at, although he is part of the group, he is in a way, a little more distant.

He is not – although he is part of the group- he is a little outsider in the group.

Okay, so let us go into his head too. And have a look at what is going on in there. That one has a kind of a headache. Okay let us get out of there Chris.

So what did you see there? Those people are doing everything to make sure you are a failure, right.

Facilitator: And can you see how they are doing that? What they are doing?

Anny: Well, acting like bachelors is about the best way I can put it, with absolutely no respect for anybody else in their lives. That is the thing. It is a very self-centred thing. They are just partying –

Here he goes again, I can see the campfire. The whole gang and laughing and beer cans. Not beer bottles, beer cans and they are laughing and so forth and so for whatever reason, that particular ad on T.V. really interests Chris. So let us go into Chris's head now and do a cleanup job here. And I can tell you…

Facilitator: And how old was he when he saw that and made an impression on him?

Anny: 16 comes up. That really impressed him. It was 16. It just came. So, I am going into his head and do a cleanup job there. I say, just a moment, this is just to sell beer. And the corporation there, that is what they want to do, sell beer. At the expense of people who are swallowing that ad.

And I am looking at Chris again and I am asking him to unhook all the hooks those supposed friends put on him to make sure he is not getting successful.

Chris, I will tell you misery loves company. Have a look at those guys. And I know they are only, you know, only 30 or about 30, but that is fine. The thing is what will happen when you are 60. Looking back.

Facilitator: What does he want to have in his life. Like what does he want to achieve, unhooking himself from his friends will make that more clear to him. What will make him happy, he himself, what is it that he wants in his life?

Anny: He wants the safety of a home. The safety of the home.

Facilitator: And when you say the safety of the home, how does he describe that?

Anny: Okay, it is the opposite of being given away... It is the opposite of being given away. So, the thing is I am looking at him here. When I say that he just about to leave... and then he comes back. Umm humm.

Anny: Okay, it is the... So is there some healing that we still need to do for him in regards to that, with his mom giving him away. He said it has to do with never being able to say no.

Anny: Yah, and you know what, how about learning to say no to your friends. To the people who call themselves your friends. How about …

Facilitator: So, what is he afraid of if he says no. What does he think would happen if he says no to some people in his life?

Anny: He does not know. He is scared.

So, all right. Well, Chris, let us see what happens. How about looking at you. What do you want in you instead of what the others want you to want?

Facilitator: Right, is he disconnected from his friends at this time?

Anny: Not yet.

Facilitator: No.

Anny: Umm umm. No, not yet. So I am... . Because he has to unhook it. I will not do it for him. Uhh uhh. Okay, there was one on him here. So, he removed that one.

Facilitator: So, as you ask him what is it that he wants will become very clear for him as he tunes into his soul, his spirit.

Anny: Chris, misery loves company.

Have a look at those guys. Have a look at how empty is their heart. How empty it is. So, okay, he is removing another one and another one was hooked here. He is removing another one, but there is another one there.

So now, Chris, if you want to be successful in life, stick around successful people. If you want to be happy in a relationship, stick around people who are very happy in a relationship and you will find that there is a way of going about it and when in a relationship, respect your mate the way you want your mate to respect you.

That is right. Imagine something. If your mate would do exactly the same thing like you, where would be the relationship, humm? Where would be the relationship? There would not be one, huh?

You are going to learn to follow your heart. Yup and am very glad that you did that now.

His cap, instead of having the thing in the back, he turned it like this. I say yah. Accept getting older and you will find that it is terrific, and I am putting something in his heart because deep down it is a lack of self-assurance really.

He is not sure of himself and deep, deep down that is what it is. So, I am putting something in there. On the picture, but with his cap like that…

Ho… because he has removed his cap and gives you a kiss. And he looks at me and he kissed the mikes. (laughter)
He looked at me and just kissed the mikes. He looked at me and said, ohhh (laughter)

Facilitator: That is it, hum.

Anny: That is it.

WRAPING IT UP WITH THE SURROGATE FOLLOWED

Feedback

I found out later the facial description of the friends was accurate.
The elusive one is the friend that indeed usually has a headache and, although part of the group, makes sure his living-in girlfriend is not aware of when he is with "the boys".

It was also confirmed that Chris always wanted to be "young" and acted like a teenager as soon as he was with a bunch of "boys".

The fact that wanted to be liked, act young and could not say NO explained how come he lets "the boys" run him by the nose.

And…
He always drinks beer in a can! He says beer in a bottle has no taste….

Facilitator's Notes – Chris' Surrogate Session

February 19th, 2004

Scared in his eyes – fear.
Very important to be popular with friends – wants to be 'liked and 'approved of' by his friends.

Fear to get older – getting older means there is no fun.
That is why he will not cut ties – girl.

Age – issue.
Staying young by staying popular with friends.

Fear – being given away (by mother).

Planning stage disposition of his soul – not being able to say 'no'.

*Not being true to himself.
Chris connected to friends – a rope is around him – what is the intent of your friend? He would do everything so Chris would lose his job and his girlfriend.

Looks into all his friend's heads – jealously – they would like to see him be a failure.
16 years old – really impressed him – 'beer commercial' – showing 'guys' all 'bonding' by a campfire and drinking the beer.

Wants the 'safety of a home' – the opposite of being given away.
Has a very hard time saying 'no'.

What does Chris want??

Question about Bruno's one-on one session

- Question 1 -

- Question 2 -

- Question 3 -

- Question 4 -

- Question 5 -

Transcript – Bruno – Motivation

Anny: What made you decide to come here? What is happening? You remember I touch your knees, do you?

Bruno: Umm. Yes. Well, basically, I have been having a lot of problems with my studies and it is more related to feelings and power flow in my body that I felt.

Anny: Is that right.

Bruno: Yah, actually it is worse than it was before. The last time I came to you, it was something similar to that. Umm and it was negative feelings and things like that. And things like me stopping me from doing things.

Anny: Yes, I remember that.

Bruno: Yah, yah.

Anny: As you talk, the whole session is coming back to me.

Bruno: Okay, and it is basically more intense now. Umm the feeling. It went away for a long time. Then we came back from Europe. Ever since then, I felt that feeling. And I am not quite too sure why.

Anny: Okay, you came back from where?

Bruno: From Europe. Yah, we went on a trip to Europe umm, during the summer.

Anny: Is that right?

Bruno: Yes.

Anny: Okay, back from Europe.

Bruno: And we went to some places that actually overwhelmed me with their feeling. Because I touch things and I can get a feeling from them. You know of bad, good, something happened here, and I entered into a lot of places that felt really familiar. I do not know if that makes a whole lot of sense, but.

Anny: Ohh, yes, you are making a lot of sense, yes.

Bruno: And umm. I touched some walls and in particular in Venice. That really bothered me and I got a lot of bad feelings from there and it is kind of…

I am not sure if that is what stuck with me or not, but I know it has been ever since we got back from Europe, I have felt very overwhelmed, very negative.

I get these really bad sensations at the back of my neck, like energy flowing from the stem of my brain, all the way to the front cerebrum into my eyes and it kind of makes me feel like my head is swimming.

Umm, and that is kind of stopping me from doing things and that kind of causes turning and twisting in my stomach because I get a bad feeling from it.

Umm, and that is stopping me from doing a lot of things and I have had a really negative outlook on things lately as a result of that. Like I am trying not to be, to be pessimistic about things and that, but it is difficult.

I am finding it ever more difficult each time that I encounter that feeling. What I am trying to get at, is that my motivation has dropped.

My …

because I feel very distressed and overwhelmed and I do not feel quite as dedicated to my studies and that as I did before and that has been a real problem as well.

Anny: Well yah. Okay.

Bruno: And I cannot seem to get over that I have been doing Reiki, I have been meditating, I have been doing you name it, you know, like trying to focus my energy.

Anny: And it is not doing a thing.

Bruno: Yah.

Anny: Okay, so now. You talked to me about your studies. What are you studying?

Bruno: Three pharmacy courses at the University.

Anny: Okay. Okay, before you went to Europe, how was it?

Bruno: Umm. Things were kind of declining very slowly.

Umm, I was feeling kind of tired at the end of the year and as a result, I was a bit lazy in my studies. But I still did very well. But it was kind of declining my feeling of dedication and that. But at the same time, it was something I could control a bit better than now. But I am feeling kind of depressed lately as well with that. Kind of lost, almost.

Anny: Okay.

Bruno: And I find lately, especially I walk into rooms and that and lights will burn out. Like there will be a flicker and it will just (zip sound) and I will hear it and I have had to change five or six lights

every time I walk into the rooms. I am not quite too sure what that is, but uhh.

Anny: Ummm.

Bruno: But I really need a solution that will last. Umm I need something that will have no time limit, no cease. You know what I mean. Something that will stay with me for good. You know what I mean?

Anny: Well of course.

Bruno: Yah, definitely so.

Anny: I wonder what happened in Europe, especially Venice, huh? I know you are married.

Bruno: Yes.

Anny: Okay, a big smile there.

Bruno: Humm humm humm.

Anny: And do you have a child?

Bruno: No.

Anny: Okay, because whoever answered the phone called you and said Grandma is calling.

Bruno: Oh no, that was my father-in-law. He thought you were my grandma. That is all. (laughter)

Anny: (laugher) I thought, maybe they have a child, you know. I am okay with that. Oh yah, I am okay with all that, it is just simply I thought well, maybe they have children.

Bruno: No, not yet.

Anny: Okay, very good. When did you marry?

Bruno: In 2001.

Anny: So you were 25.

Bruno: That is right.

Anny: How old was she?

Bruno: Same age.

Anny: Same age. And what is her first name?

Bruno: Rosa.

Anny: Rosa, Okay. (cough). All right, so here you are.

Bruno: Also, there is another problem. **I am finding that forever reason, my memory retention is not what it used to be for some reason. I do not understand why. That was never a problem before.** In fact, all of my teachers always commented that I had such a good memory and actually it was photographic before. But **now I cannot seem to retain any information** and it is also, I kind of think it is attributed to that feeling too. Because I open up my textbooks and instantly, I get that feeling. **Instantly, that overwhelmed negative feeling and I am reading things and as I read it, I forget it.**

Anny: Well yah, oh yah.
Bruno: And I do not understand why. I really do not understand it. But I really need help with that as well.

Anny: Well you have to fix that all right.

Bruno: Because I keep, you know,

I will – I will – I will read something over and I will do what I used to do. I will read over 5 or 6 times and just like look away and say it in my head. And I will move on a couple pages and then I will come across that term again and I will be like, what does that mean.

I do not remember what that means and then I will have to go back and its very slow moving right now.

Anny: All right, umm humm.   Okay, Bruno, be prepared for anything and I mean anything.   Okay, because you are giving me information there that is umm humm…

Okay, very good, I have a good idea what it is. And for you, just be prepared for anything and be comfortable with it.

Bruno: Okay.

Anny: Okay, because something happened that is for sure. Okay.

Bruno: Okay.

Anny: So you went to Italy or to Europe?

Bruno: We went to all of Europe. We went to, well a lot of it anyway, not all. Umm, France, Spain, Italy, Greece and on the way back, we went to London, so.

Anny: That must have been quite a pleasant trip, huh.
Bruno: It was. Yes.

Anny: You liked that, did you not?

Bruno: Oh it was a lot of fun.

Anny: And how was Rosa? How did she like that?

Bruno: She enjoyed a lot as well. Yah.

Anny: She did.

Bruno: She misses it a lot.

Anny: She misses it?

Bruno: Yes she does.

Anny: How come?

Bruno: She really enjoys travelling a lot.

Anny: Humm?

Bruno: She really enjoys travelling a lot.

Anny: Which is great.

Bruno: Yes, yes, definitely.

Anny: Which is great.

Bruno: Yah, but she misses the experiencing things every day. Something new every day and now it is kind of back to routine and it is kind of a drag for her.

Anny: Okay, all right. Very good. So you have been married five years now.

Bruno: That is right.

Anny: Time goes by fast, huh?

Bruno: It does. Yes.

Anny: First thing you say, what happened.

Bruno: (laughter)

Anny: So first thing you know, 50 years later, you say, what happened. That is about the size of it.

Bruno: Yah.

Anny: Okay, humm. (cough)

Stare at my fingers and listen to my voice. Keep your gaze on my fingers and listen to my voice. That is right. Just keep your gaze on my fingers and listen to my voice. Take a slow deep breath and as you exhale, close your eyes.

And enjoy the experience. Enjoy the relaxation and during this session, each time I am clearing my throat, you will go so much deeper. So much deeper into relaxation (cough).

Deeper and deeper. Deeper and deeper and deeper. And become aware of your lungs. Your lungs. They are expanding and contracting. Expanding and contracting in a beautiful rhythmic manner. And every breath you take makes you go deeper and deeper,

and deeper into relaxation and as your breath flows. As it comes, as it goes, notice that the sensation is a little cooler when you breath in, than when you breath out. Just a little cooler, and the familiar sounds of this room make you so relaxed.

So comfortable. So relaxed. So comfortable. Letting all your cares fade away, fade away, fade away, fade away.

As I am asking for your protection and well being. And I say God, please allow only good things to come to Bruno, and to me Anny, the hypnotherapist.

And for this blessing, we give thanks.

And now, you ask to be placed into the protection of your very own light. Your very own light, your spark of life. It is like a mini sun in your chest. Some people can see it, some people can feel it, some people simply know it is there. That light of yours, that very beautiful light of yours. Let it shine, let it shine, let it shine throughout every cell of your body. Throughout your aura. Cleansing your body, cleansing your aura. Strengthening your body, strengthening your aura. Extending itself at one arm's length above you, beneath you, at each side of you, in front of you and behind you and mentally repeat with me. This is my body, this my space. Only light can come to me. Only light can come from me. Only my light can be here.

And as you take a slow deep breath and exhale, sleep now. Inhale, slowly exhale. Sleep now. When I say sleep now, this is not the sleep you experience when you fall asleep at night. I am talking about what is called the hypnotic sleep. This means you relax completely your mind and your body, so your subconscious mind freed of all restrain is open and receptive to the suggestions you are receiving during this session and during this session the sound of my voice will make you go deeper and deeper and deeper into relaxation. During this session, each time I am touching one of your knees, you will go twice as deep into relaxation and also during this session, each time the ventilation system is going on and off, on and off, you will go so much deeper, so much deeper into relaxation. And now, find yourself at a time on your trip when you felt…

Go to the beginning of the trip. Feeling absolutely great. Happy to be there. Finding it interesting, fascinating and comfortable. And when you are there, let me know.

Bruno: (nod)

Anny: All right, breath in that feeling. Just breath it in and enjoy it. Enjoy it. Just breath it in. Breathing that feeling. That is right. That is right. And now, as you take a

slow deep breath and exhale, you are going to advance to something changed and you start to feel…

There is something that happened there and you feel negative.

The first thing that comes to you. Just advance to when all of a sudden something – you could just feel it. You felt overwhelmed and you have some very, very negative feeling. The first thing (click of fingers) that came to you.

Bruno: Bordeaux

Anny: Bordeaux. Overwhelmed. What is happening there? How do you feel? What happened in Bordeaux?

Bruno: I feel annoyed.

Anny: Say that again.

Bruno: **I feel annoyed.**

Anny: **Feeling annoyed. Feeling annoyed** huh. All right. I would like you to go back and forth on your trip from then on and become very much aware of what is going on there. Hey, you are **feeling annoyed** are you not?

Bruno: Umm humm.

Anny: **Feeling annoyed.** With each inhale, allow that **annoyed feeling** to come to you stronger and stronger and stronger and I know you do not like it. For now just allow it to be there and with each exhale, find yourself going back, back, back to the same feeling in another situation. Trust what comes. (coughing) Whatever comes to you.

Bruno: We are in Neconos.

Anny: Humm?

Bruno: We are in Neconos.

Anny: And where is that?

Bruno: In the Greek Islands.

Anny: And what is happening that you **feel annoyed** again.

Bruno: It is not what we expected at all.

Anny: Ohh, **feeling annoyed** huh. **Feeling annoyed. Feeling annoyed. Feeling annoyed.** I would like you to pay attention to your body. When you **feel annoyed** like that, where does it sit in your body?

Bruno: In my stomach.

Anny: Put your hands on it, both. Yah, it is important for the feeling to know you know it is there. And it is **feeling annoyed. Feeling annoyed.** And as you take a slow deep breath and exhale, mentally go into the **annoyed feeling.** Just mentally go into that **annoyed feeling** and according to that **annoyed feeling**, how old are you. Go deep down there. Go into the **annoyed feeling.** How old?

Bruno: 56

Anny: You are 56. All right. And what is your name?

Bruno: John

Anny: I did not get that.

Bruno: John.

Anny: John, John. John is 56 and he is **feeling annoyed**. John is **feeling annoyed,** and he is 56. And as you take a slow deep breath and exhale, I would like John to let us know what is it that he is **feeling annoyed** like that? What is happening that John is annoyed? Trust what comes. Totally trust what comes.

Bruno: Work is not going well.

Anny: What is not going well?

Bruno: Work.

Anny: Work is not going well. Humm. Take a deep breath and as you exhale, I am asking John to make you aware of what was not going well at work. I would like John to make you aware of what was happening that things are not going well at work. And totally trust what comes.

Bruno: He lost a lot of money.

Anny: Lost a lot of money. And how does that feel?

Bruno: Very disappointing.

Anny: Umm humm. Take a deep breath Bruno and as you exhale, I am asking John to make you aware of what type of work it was. What type of work it was that he lost money?

Bruno: Bank owner.

Anny: Humm?

Bruno: Bank owner.

Anny: Bank owner. Umm humm. For a bank owner losing a lot of money is not exactly what a bank is for, huh. And I understand John very well here. And as you take a slow deep breath and exhale, I would like to know what is it that – at what point did John join Bruno? And go back and forth and back and forth. There is a point where John decided.

Bruno: Paris.

Anny: Paris, okay. All right and I would like John to explain to me what was it that he decides that it gets to be going along with Bruno. What was it? There was something about Bruno.

Bruno: He was worried about the trip.

Anny: Bruno was worried about the trip?

Bruno: Yes.

Anny: Okay. So what was the idea of joining Bruno. What was it for? What was the intent here? Trust what comes.

Bruno: To help.

Anny: To help, yahh. Ummm humm. Well thank you very much John. Now there is one thing I would like to know. Do you remember when you had your own bank, when you had your own body and everything? Do you remember that time?

Bruno: No.

Anny: You do not? What was the highlight of your life John? What was the highlight?

Bruno: My wife.

Anny: My wife. Is that right. Your wife, huh. And what country – in what country did you have your bank.

Or… you know… you know… I have no idea,… it was a banker who was travelling a lot. I have no idea… So I would like you to tell me John, what was your main country of business.

Bruno: America.

Anny: Where?

Bruno: America.

Anny: America, is that right. And what were you doing in Paris?

Bruno: Travelling.

Anny: I did not get that.

Bruno: Travelling.

Anny: Travelling, yahh. It makes sense, does it not. So, umm humm…
John just take some slow deep breath and as you exhale, just relax, just relax, just relax and remember the highlights of your life. What pleased you the most. Just remember that John, and relax and as you relax, Bruno is relaxing too.

And as you take a slow deep breath, both of you. As you exhale, John go back to the end of your life as a banker. Go back there. The end of your life as a banker. And tell me how old were you?

Bruno: 62

Anny: Humm?

Bruno: 62

Anny: 62. 62, is that right. 62 years old. And how does it feel as you are going… You could feel that you are going to the end of your life. How did it feel?

Bruno: Depressed.

Anny: You felt depressed. What is it that you were feeling depressed about?

Bruno: I was leaving too early.

Anny: I was leaving too early. All right. And as you take a slow deep breath and exhale now, you are about to die, you are about to die John. You are about to die, you are about to die John. What is going on? How did you feel?

Bruno: Desperate.

Anny: Umm humm. Very desperate. And what was going on as you are desperate? What was going on as you were desperate?
Bruno: I do not want to leave.

Anny: You do not want to leave. All right. So now as you take a slow deep breath and exhale, your body is dead now. Your body is dead. You are out of the body. You are out of the body. Your body is dead and you do not want to leave. Your body is dead. Turn around and have a look at that body of yours. Where are you, what is going on?

Bruno: I am in the street.

Anny: What did you say?

Bruno: I am in the street.

Anny: You are in the street, yahhh. And what is going on with your body? You left your body.

Bruno: People are standing around me.

Anny: Umm humm and you are in the street huh?

Bruno: Yes.

Anny: How did it feel?

Bruno: Embarrassing.

Anny: It was embarrassing. What was embarrassing?

Bruno: Everyone saw me that way.

Anny: Is that right. All right. Now John, have you ever thought you could have your bank again? In your bank, have you ever thought about that?

Bruno: No

Anny: Would you like to be in business again and this time with the experience you gained you will be very successful at it.

Bruno: Yah.

Anny: All right. John, do you trust me?

Bruno: Yes.

Anny: Thank you John. Here is what I m suggesting to you.

You can see Bruno do you?

I would like you to clean up your room so to speak. Because you have been with Bruno. Some things of yours's with Bruno now. So what I would like you to do is clean up your room so to speak. Everything that belongs to you that you put in Bruno – everything, I would like you to take it back. Because where you are going to go, you need everything that belongs to you. That is right. With your emotion, the depression, the desperation, the annoyance, you name it, everything that belongs to you. Physical sensations, you name it, everything that belongs to you. I would like you to take it out of Bruno's body and out of Bruno's energy field and put it in suitcases and since you have been travelling lately, you know the type of suitcases. It is not suitcases. It is quite fancy luggage, right. Get yourself some brand new luggage and put all your stuff in those very nice and comfortable luggage. And when he is finished Bruno, let me know.

Bruno: (nod)

Anny: Thank you. **So now, Bruno, I would like you to have your light shine with all its might to flush out whatever residues have to be flushed out and whatever residue that belongs to John, have it in his suitcase too. It is important that he is complete. So just let that…, your light shine with all its might. Flushing out whatever residue, the negative feelings, the desperation, the depression. Everything, everything that belongs to John. It belongs to John, so give it back to him and when you are finished, let me know.**

Bruno: (nod)

Anny: Thank you. **So now, Bruno, have a look at John and you are going to notice that John is standing on the pathway made of light and I would like you to help John walk on that pathway.**

John, you are going to go towards the light and that light is like a highway so to speak. A highway home. Your very own home and at that place you will be able to choose the perfect country for you. Everything that is perfect for you, so whatever career you want to embark next time, you will be born in that country. Everything is going to go well for you and maybe as you are going home through that highway of light, maybe you will even meet your wife again. Maybe she is waiting there. I do not know. That you will have to find out. And when you are both in front of that doorway or that gate, that highway so to speak, let me know Bruno.

Bruno: (nod)

Anny: So now, John, any suggestions you want to give Bruno so that he is successful in what you would like him to be successful at? Tell him now and when he is finished, let me know.

Bruno: (nod)

Anny: Thank you. So now Bruno, any recommendation you want to make John so that he has a wonderful trip back home with all of his luggage or whatever else you want to tell him, just tell him now.

Bruno: (nod)

Anny: Thank you. So now, make sure you put the luggage first on that highway so to speak and <u>help John go through that light </u>and when he is gone, let me know.

Bruno: (nod)

Anny: And now Bruno, become aware of your light again. That light of yours. Let it shine in all its might. All that cleansed space is your very own energy. And when it is done, simply nod.

Bruno: (nod)

Anny: Thank you. And as you take a slow deep breath and exhale, I would like you to check your aura. And you will know where your aura, your energy field… you will know where John was either attached, or whatever. You are going to know. And totally trust it and when you got that spot, let me know.

Bruno: (nod)

Anny: All right. Have a good look at your energy field Bruno and repair it. Sew it back with gold thread. Repair that spot. Repair it. Sew it back together. Rearrange it so it is nice and even all over you. And totally trust what is coming to your awareness. And when it is done, let me know.

Bruno: (nod)

Anny: Thank you. And now Bruno, look back into your own life and find yourself at one of the most exciting and wonderful time in your present life.
Yah, and breath in that feeling. Just breath it in. That is right. Just breath it in. Just breath it in. Just breath in your very own pleasure. Your very own energy. Your very, very own energy. Very, very own energy.

As something inside of you has shifted and your subconscious mind open and very receptive to the suggestions you are receiving now is making all the necessary adjustment right now. So that you feel great. You feel at peace. You have excellent, excellent memory recall. Great motivation, feeling absolutely wonderful. Full of energy, at peace with yourself and with the world around you. That is right, at peace with the world and yourself.

Feeling so great, so great and the benefits of this session will stay with you for hours, days, weeks, months, and years to come. And so it is. And so it is.

And bless your light. The spark of life you have within you. And thank God, whoever you perceive God to be for the wonders of life. And when you are ready Bruno, you will take a slow deep breath, open your eyes and give yourself a nice stretch. Anything surprise.

Bruno: Yah.

Anny: Okay.

Bruno: I feel a bit lighter now.

Anny: You are feeling what?

Bruno: Lighter.

Anny: Oh yes you will, absolutely.

Bruno: Umm.

Anny: A session like this, many people go back on the scale after this and they are lighter. Umm humm. Yahh. ….
Any questions or anything?

Bruno: Did something cling onto me?

Anny: Yup.

Bruno: Humm.

Anny: And you gave me the hint when you say that light bulbs are burning out with a sound, I knew.

Bruno: Humm.

Anny: I call that psychic interference, but there are many names for that. Yah, and you are feeling lighter all right.

Bruno: Umm humm.

Anny: Okay. And that is it for today. Don't you think so?

Bruno: Umm humm.

Anny: **And there is one thing though and I will leave the tape on here to explain that to you. Understand that after something like this, there is quite an energy shift in you, which is normal. Because it was all energy. So, be very careful what you are eating for the next 3 days. Listen to your body. Well listen always to your body, but specially at the moment because your body has to readjust. So when you start to eat and you feel uhhh, just stop it immediately. Just stop immediately. Whatever you eat or drink.**

Bruno: Okay.

Anny: Yup, just pay close attention. You drink and then you feel. Is your body okay with that for now.

Bruno: Okay.

Anny: Umm humm. It takes about 2 or 3 days and it is a totally normal thing. It is your body readjusting at your very own energy. Okay. You look amused now. All right. So who was annoyed at Bordeaux, in Venice and in the Greek Islands?

Bruno: Yah, that was not me.

Anny: That was not you, yah. All right.

Question about Susan's one-on one session

- Question 1 -

- Question 2 -

- Question 3 -

- Question 4 -

- Question 5 -

Transcript – Suzanne – One On One Session

February 2003

Anny: Okay Suzanne. So tell me about the whole situation there. What is happening. You could not breathe, but there is something also about… … what does that have to do with the darkness and your fear of the darkness?

Suzanne: The darkness is really connected. I was thinking about that last night and if it is not dark, I am okay. Like I can be in a small, small space. Elevators. Anything, it does not bother me. It is the darkness. It is more the darkness, I guess. I used to be afraid of the dark as a child too.

Anny: Is that right?

Suzanne: (laugh)

A: Tell me about it. Put your hand (Client spontaneously put her hand on her heart) … that is okay. Tell me about it. You were scared of the dark too when you were a little girl.

Suzanne: Yah.

Anny: Tell me about it.

Suzanne: Humm. I do not know. I was just always afraid of the dark and **I wanted** the light on. Or **some light.**

Anny: **You wanted some light.**

Suzanne: Yah. Afraid of something in my closest. Afraid of something under my bed. I do not know.

Anny: And what was happening?

Suzanne: I used to sleep walk.

Anny: You did.

Suzanne: And I used to leave the house and I used to go out in the woods. And the only way I know that, is that I overheard my Mom telling somebody one day and that really scared me.

Anny: I can hear it in your voice. You can feel it just talking about it.

Suzanne: Because I was afraid of the dark and to think that I was outside. We lived in a trailer court in the middle of the woods and so I go off in the woods. And I mean, just the thought of that, oh my goodness.

Anny: And what would happen when you… You should feel yourself, you are trembling.

Suzanne: I do not know. She just said I would be knocking at the door at four in the morning to come back in. I have no idea. I do not remember anything other than I would get up and leave the house and go for a walk in my pyjamas in the woods and come back and knock at the door.

Anny: And how old were you then?

Suzanne: Before school. Let us see. I would have to – probably maybe five when we lived there.

Anny: How many brothers and sisters do you have?

Suzanne: One sister, one brother.

Anny: What is the age difference? How many years younger or how many years older?

Suzanne: My **sister is 14 months older.**

Anny: Your **sister is 14 months older.**

Suzanne: And my brother. He must be. He was adopted. He must be eight years younger. I think.

Anny: Okay.

Suzanne: Something like that.

Anny: Now. If I remember well from other sessions, there was something about your father leaving right?

Suzanne: Yup.

Anny: You are the one?

Suzanne: Yah, my biological Father when I was about two I think. Somewhere in there.

Anny: And I do not remember something about – did your Mother remarry?

Suzanne: Umm humm.

Anny: How old were you then?

Suzanne: Ohhh. You know I do not know cause she never told us when they got married. It was never said, even after he died and they never celebrated anniversaries. But I would say, I can remember him being there when I was just before we moved to the ManTech Dam. That is where all this happened. So I must have been four or five. Somewhere in there.

Anny: When he moved in?

Suzanne: Yah. When they got married. I think they got married. Probably four. I do not know. Four.

Anny: And the sleep walking that you are aware of happened after.

Suzanne: Yahh, **yahhhh.**

Anny: How did it feel to say **yahhhh?**

Suzanne: (laugh)

Anny: **How did it feel?**

Suzanne: **Actually, actually a sense of relief. And I do not know why?**

Anny: **No questions asked.**

Suzanne: Well I do know actually.

Anny: **What is it?**

Suzanne: **Because, because somewhere inside said it was not because of my (laugh) father. Was not because of my, who I consider my real father. Because it was after that.**

Anny: Okay.

Suzanne: I do not know. I mean not. I do not know, maybe it did. But I just got relief because suddenly it was like ohh it was not right when he moved in, it was after. Because we were very close.

Anny: All right. Now, tell me about – you said it was in a trailer park in the middle of the woods.

Suzanne: Yahh, there was about 100 trailers and it was uhhh, at the ManTech Dam, which is about… It was kind of a camp and people lived there for about two or three years.

Anny: (coughing) Umm humm. Oh yah.

Suzanne: And they built the ManTech Dam, so we had kind of like a bunk house, confectionery and a little movie hall. All trailers.

Anny: Yes, I am quite familiar with all that stuff.

Suzanne: Yah, and you know, in the middle of the bush. And I did not even like going in there in the day time. Kids would go in there and play and I just felt like they should not be out there. For some reason I just thought they were trespassing in the woods. And it was not a place to be, so it really bothered me when I found out I was doing that anyway.

Anny: Okay, now how old were you when your parents moved there?

Suzanne: Must have been five. It was the year before I started school. It was, let me think. You know I must have been six when this was happening. I think. I do not know. It was just before I started school, we moved there.

Anny: Okay.

Suzanne: And my birthday is in March, so, I think I must have been six then, when we moved there.

Anny: And when did you start the sleep walking?

Suzanne: Grade 4, so that's when we moved. But, uhh, it was some… I don't know. I think it was within that first year we lived there. But I really don't know.

Anny: Okay. Very good. Fair enough. How does it feel there now?, (where client had her hand)

Suzanne: (laugh) Shaky. I do not know.

Anny: It feels.

Suzanne: Yah, a little bit. It feels better with my hand there. It feels like I am pushing it down. Actually, yah, that is what it feels like when I am holding it there.

Anny: Okay, how about being kind to it.

Suzanne: Ahh, okay.

Anny: What I would like to know, is it possible for you to go inside that feeling there and ask that feeling how old were you when it came to you?

Suzanne: (laugh) Okay. (heavy breath)

Anny: That is right, how old was Suzanne when that feeling came to her?

Suzanne: In this life you mean?

Anny: How old was Suzanne when that feeling came to Suzanne? Totally trust what comes and as you are connecting with it, you are feeling yourself becoming more and more relaxed. More and more at peace. Letting all your cares fade away, fade away, fade away.

Deepening the trance within a time frame
And the familiar sounds of this room make you so relaxed. So comfortable and during this experience, each time I am clearing my throat you become more and more relaxed. More and more (cough) relaxed.

Asking for protection

As I am asking (clear throat) (cough) for your protection and well being and I say, God, please allow only good things to come to Suzanne and, to me Anny, the hypnotherapist. And for this blessing, we give thanks. (Coughing)

And now you ask to be placed into the protection of your very own light. Your very own light. Your spark of life. It is like a mini sun in your chest. Some people can feel it. Some people can see it. Some people simply know it is there. That light of yours. That very beautiful light of yours, let it shine. Let it shine. Let it shine throughout every cell of your body. Throughout your aura. Cleansing your body. Cleansing your aura. Strengthening your body. Strengthening your aura. Extending itself at one arm's length above you, beneath you, at each side of you, in front of you and behind you and mentally repeat with me. This is my body, this is my space. Only light can come to me. Only light can come from me. Only my light can be here.

Suggestions within a time frame
And during this session, each time you inhale, the feelings are coming to you stronger and stronger and with each exhale, you find yourself going all the way, all the way back to where that feeling comes from.

Checking where the feeling is coming from/who's feeling is it.
So as you are having your hand on that feeling with each exhale, you find yourself going all the way back to whatever it is that started that feeling. Totally trust what comes to you and when you have it let me know. That feeling in your chest, be kind to it. There is a feeling there. A feeling. What is it, trust what comes.

Suzanne: What is the feeling?

Anny: Umm humm. Where does it come from? Trust what comes.

Suzanne: Confinement. There is **a sense of confinement.**

Anny: **A sense of confinement. A sense of confinement.**
With each inhale, that **sense of confinement** is going to come to you stronger and stronger and I know you do not like it. Just stay with it for

now. The feeling wants to tell you something. So with each inhale that **sense of confinement** is coming to you stronger and stronger and stronger. And with each exhale, you find yourself going all the way back to one of the first time you have, had a **sense of confinement.** Whatever it is, just go there. Allow yourself to go all the way to the beginning of that **sense of confinement.** Go back there. Trust what comes.

Suzanne: I do not know. I am, I am, I do not know where. I am. There is, **I do not know where I am at.**

Anny: **You do not know where you are at,** and?

Suzanne: There is dirt or **dust falling**. I do not know.

Anny: **Dust falling**. All right. Take a deep breath and as you exhale, look down at your feet. Where are you?

Suzanne: **There is some sand.**

Anny: **There is some sand.**

Suzanne: **Bare feet.**

Anny: **Bare feet.**

Suzanne: It is **like a tomb.**

Anny: **Like a tomb. Sand.** And as you are looking at your feet. Your **bare feet**. What gender are you? Trust what comes. Totally trust what comes.

Suzanne: They look like men.

Anny: All right.

Suzanne: Men's feet. They are wide.

Anny: All right. So (cough), as you take a slow deep breath and exhale, you are going to rewind the movie of time. Rewind the movie of time. All the way back to when you felt quite comfortable. And when you are there, let me know. It felt comfortable. Way back. Just rewind the movie of time. Rewind it. All the way back to when it felt comfortable.

Suzanne: **I am laughing.**

Anny: **You're laughing**. And what is going on?

Suzanne: **I am laying on cushions** of some kind, laughing.

Anny: **You are laying on cushions**. And how do you feel?

Suzanne: Good.

Anny: Umm humm.

Suzanne: Happy. **In charge,** I do not know.

Anny: Ummm? I did not get that.

Suzanne: **In charge.**

Anny: You feel **in charge.** How does it feel to be **in charge**?

Suzanne: **Normal.**

Anny: **It feels normal.**

Suzanne: **I have everything I need.**

Anny: **You had everything you need and you are laughing.**

Feel that laughter within you. Just feel that laughter. And as you are feeling that laughter, you are going deeper and deeper in a very special quality of relaxation. Deeper and deeper, deeper and deeper and deeper and as you take a slow deep breath (inhale) and exhale, you are going to advance to whatever it is that got you in that place that gave you **a sense of confinement.** Just before – there is something about it. Whatever it is that got you to have that **sense of confinement**. What is happening? Trust what comes, even if it doesn't make sense to you.

Suzanne: **I have broken the law.**

Anny: **You have broken the law**. And? And?

Suzanne: And, **that was the punishment.**

Anny: And **that was the punishment**. And what **was the punishment?**

Suzanne: **To be entombed.**

Anny: **To be entombed.** Take a deep breath and as you exhale, you are going to rewind the movie of time to just before you find out **you broke the law**. And trust what comes.

Suzanne: Umm.

Anny: And how do you feel?

Suzanne: **I feel, like I can do anything.**

Anny: **You feel like you can do anything.**

Suzanne: Yahh, because there is something. I am, I do not know. **I can do anything** because I am wealthy and I am one of those who have.

Anny: Because you're wealthy and you are one of those.

Suzanne: Yah, and we had power.

Anny: Okay, very good.

As too much emotions are coming up, asking client to be an observer.
So now, as you take a slow deep breath and exhale, you will find yourself looking at the whole situation. You will be watching the whole thing unfold. How did that person get into the tomb? Trust what comes.

Suzanne: I thought I could do anything.

Anny: And then, what happened next?

Suzanne: I could not. I found out I did not have that power.

Anny: You did not have that power. And then what happened next?

Suzanne: They put me in a tomb, dragging and screaming.

Anny: Who are they?

Suzanne: **Two people.**

Anny: **Two people.**

Suzanne: They were not anybody. Just people.

Anny: Then, describe me as you are observing everything how did that man get into the tomb?

Suzanne: He was **thrown in.**

Anny: **Thrown in**. And then what happened next?

Suzanne: **Forcefully.**

Anny: **Forcefully**, and then what happened next?

Suzanne: **They closed it off.**

Anny: **They closed it off .**

Suzanne: **And now the sand is falling.**

Anny: **And the sand is falling**. And what happened next? They closed it off, and?

Suzanne: **It is darkness.**

Anny: **It is darkness.**

Asking client to go to the end quickly
All right. Take a slow deep breath and as you exhale, you are going to advance to… all the way to when the end of whatever it was. Advance to the end of it quickly.

Suzanne: (breath)

Anny: Get back to the end of it.

Suzanne: (whispering) **I cannot breath.**

Anny: **You cannot breath.** What is happening that **you cannot breathe?**

Suzanne: There is no air. (gasping for breath)

Anny: All right.

Asking client to move to the end quickly
So, take a deep breath and as you exhale, you are out of your body now. Out of your body. And what was going on that you are out of your body?

Suzanne: (whisper) **It is quiet.**

Anny: **It is quiet.**

Suzanne: **Calm.**

Anny: And **calm**. And as you are looking at your body, give me a description of it. What do you see?

Suzanne: I was wearing blue with gold. It is like **a soldier's outfit.**

Anny: **A soldier's outfit.**

Suzanne: It is like **Roman times.**

Anny: **Roman times.**

Suzanne: That is what it reminds me of. Rome or Egypt. Rome I think.

Anny: And how do you feel as you are looking at it?

Suzanne: **Relieved.**

Anny: **Relieved.**
As you have that feeling of relief, you will find your hand is getting so heavy that it is gently sliding on your lap as you go deeper and deeper and deeper into relaxation. And what happened next? What happened next?

Suzanne: **It is quiet.**

Anny: Ummm?

Suzanne: (whisper) **It is quiet.**

Anny: **It is quiet**. And then what happened next?

Suzanne: (breath)

Anny: Trust what comes. What happened next? **It is quiet, relief, it is quiet,** what happened next?

Suzanne: (whisper) I am just kind of **looking around.**

Anny: Humm?

Suzanne: **Looking around at everything.**

Anny: And what is it about it that you **look around at everything.**

Suzanne: **Kind of reviewing all of it.**

Anny: Umm humm.

Suzanne: What happened and why.

Anny: Umm humm.
So take a deep breath and as you exhale, I would like you to review what happened that you got thrown into that tomb. What happened that you got thrown into that tomb?

Suzanne: Well thinking I was really powerful.

Anny: Yah, and?

Suzanne: And nothing could touch me.

Anny: Yes, and?

Suzanne: **And overstepping the bounds**.

Anny: **Overstepping your bounds.**

Suzanne: Yahh.

Anny: And what is it – whose boundaries. Who established those boundaries? Where does those boundaries come from? Trust what comes

Suzanne: The people.

Anny: And then what happened next?

Suzanne: Humm. **They over threw me.**

Anny: **They over threw you.**

Suzanne: Umm humm.

Anny: All right. **So here you are now reviewing everything.**

Suzanne: Umm humm.

Checking to know whose past life is it
Anny: And what happened next?

Suzanne: Then they threw me in the tomb.

Anny: Yah.

Suzanne: Shut the door of it. They were rocks.

Anny: Umm humm.

Suzanne: A big rock. It took a lot of them.

Anny: Umm humm. And then what happened next.

Suzanne: I died.

Anny: And then after that, what happened next? Trust what comes.

Suzanne: **I reviewed everything for a while.**

Anny: **You reviewed everything for a while.**

Suzanne: Yah.

Anny: And then?

Suzanne: And then I learned about power.

Anny: What is that?

Suzanne: Real power – what that was. (big breath)

Anny: Tell me about it.

Suzanne: About controls.

Anny: How did you find out about that?

Suzanne: (breath) From those who were wiser than me.

Anny: All right.

Suzanne: I do not know who.

Anny: That is all right.
Take a deep breath and as you exhale in your mind, join that man in the tomb.
And explain to him how we got to him. Same **feelings**. **Feeling of confinement** in the chest and ask him if he would be willing to help you with something and what is his answer?

Suzanne: With what?

Anny: With that. First of all, how does he want me to call him?

Finding whose past life it is.
Suzanne: Jacob.

Anny: Jacob?

Suzanne: That is what I heard. I do not know.

Anny: That is fine. Just trust what comes. Jacob. Okay Jacob.

Explain to him that we connect with him by following your feelings about the darkness and a sense of confinement. And tell him how did you get those feelings from him? We are in 2003 – how did you get those feelings from him?
Trust what comes. Jacob will know – Jacob knows.

Suzanne: Cause he died in panic.

Anny: Because he died in panic, and?

Suzanne: He could not breath.

Anny: And could not breathe. That is right.

Suzanne: Or see.

Anny: Or see, yahh. Ask him did he ever get to a time after that where he could see the light? He could see the daylight.

Suzanne: Umm humm.

Anny: By with his mind going out of that tomb. He could see the daylight.

Suzanne: It was awhile first, but he could.

Anny: Ohh, ask him what is it about it that it took him awhile?

Suzanne: He calmed down. He needed to calm down.

Confirming whose past life client accessed.

Anny: Is that right. **So ask him at what point did you start to have his feelings? Ask him at what point did you start to have his feelings?**

Suzanne: Of calm?

Anny: No, of the way he felt about the darkness and the breathing and put your hand on your chest again so he knows what feelings you are talking about. That feeling there. Because he was in that tomb and he could not breath, plus the panic because he could not see.

Suzanne: When the rock came across and shut.

Anny: Right. You understand that don you? Right. So ask him, what is it about you that you got the same feeling as him? Ask him. How old were you when that feeling came to you? Trust what comes.

Suzanne: Do you mean in this life?

Anny: Umm humm. Ask him and totally trust what comes. Even if it does not make sense at all. At what point did it become your feelings?

Suzanne: In the womb.

Anny: In the womb. Is that right? So ask – what was it about the womb that you started to have those feelings?

Suzanne: It was dark and confining.

Anny: It was dark and confining.

Suzanne: I could not breath, yah.

Anny: Yah. You understand that don't you? So now, ask him to have a look at you. Does he know that you are out of there? So what is it – what is it that you still got that feeling? Ask him. Ask him what is his fear that he still feels confined and cannot breath. What is it that he still feels that way? Ask him. Trust what comes.

Suzanne: Getting closed off.

Anny: I did not get that.

Suzanne: (clear throat) Feeling closed off.

Anny: Closed off from what? Ask him.

Suzanne: It is a feeling of not knowing the way out. I do not know.

Anny: Not knowing the way out. You understand that don't you. Yah, tell him. Tell Jacob that you understand. Ask him would he like to have some help so that he finds his way out? So, ask him.

Suzanne: He wants to be free.

Clearing client

Anny: He wants to be free. All right. As Jacob wants to be free, we find again your hand become extremely heavy and sliding down to your lap. And ask Jacob to have a look at you and take out of your system everything. All the feelings that belongs to him and put it in bags, so to speak. Just like luggage bags from Roman time. And put them in bags that are on your right-hand side. And you will become very much aware of what he's taking out of you. Ask him to take everything that belongs to him out of your system and when he's done, let me know. (music)

Suzanne: Okay.

Anny: I am addressing myself to you now. You are going to help him get out of the situation. He wants to be free. And for that, we need his help. Thatis the reason I ask him to take everything that belongs to him. All the fears, the feelings – everything out of your system and put it in bags on your right hand side. Because the setting free, it is important that he takes everything that belongs to him with him. And I would like

Jacob to let me know what is that he liked the most when he had a body? What is it that he liked the most? What was great to be alive? And I would like to know what it is.

Suzanne: He liked his physical body and experiencing things.

Anny: All right. Now I am asking something to Jacob. Whatever decision he made about power and money as he was dying in that tomb, I am asking Jacob to make sure he takes all those decisions about money and power out of your system too. They are his and put it in bags on your left-hand side. When he is finished, let me know.

Suzanne: It is done.

Sending the Entity to the light
Anny: So now, Jacob wants to be set free. As you are observing Jacob, you will notice that he is standing on a pathway made of light. Ask him to come along with you to the light up above and make sure he takes all his luggage with him – it is his. And when you are both in front of that light up above, let me know.

Suzanne: Umm humm.

Anny: So now, ask Jacob, what is it about you that he was attracted to you?

Suzanne: About me?

Anny: Yahh. Trust what comes, even if it doesn't make sense to you.
Suzanne:: Strong will power.

Anny: Umm?

Suzanne: My will.

Anny: Your will. Very good. Anything you wish to tell Jacob before he goes through the light? When you are finished, let me know.

Suzanne: Umm humm.

Anny: All right. Now Jacob expressed his wish to be set free. So as you take a slow deep breath and exhale, help him through the light and make sure he got all his luggage with him. And when he is gone, let me know.

Suzanne: Umm.

Healing client's energy field.
Anny: Thank you. And now that light of yours, that very beautiful light of yours, let it shine, let it shine in all its might. Filling all the place that were cleansed. Filling it up with your own energy and at the same time flushing out whatever has to be flushed out of there. Fill up your own space with your own energy and extend it at one arm's length above you, beneath you, at each side of you, in front of you and behind you. And mentally repeat with me, this is my body. This is my space. Only light can come to me. Only light can come from me. Only my light can be here. And breath in easily. That is right. And how do you feel now? How do you feel?

Suzanne: Free.

Wrapping it up with client. Closure.
Anny: You feel free. That feeling free feeling – breathe it in. Just breathe it in. That is right. Just breathe it in. And bless each member of your household. Bless your family. Bless your friends. Bless your pets if you have any and that includes your houseplants. Bless your possessions. And bless your wishes. Thank Jacob to have chosen freedom. Bless your light. That spark of life that you have within you and thank God, whoever you perceive God to be for the wonders of life. As your subconscious mind open and very, very receptive to the suggestions you are receiving now is making all the necessary changes

right now. That from now on, you feel comfortable. Feeling free. Breathing easily.

Honouring whatever client did to heal, prior to this session.
And the benefits of this session and the benefit of all the counselling you had prior to this session will stay with you for hours, days, weeks, months and years to come and so it is. And so it is. And your subconscious mind, open and very receptive to the suggestions you are receiving now will keep sorting all things out and will reveal to you whatever it feels you should know and understand about your feelings. And the information will come to you at most unexpected times, much to your surprise and delight. So just relax. Just relax and let all your cares fade away. Fade away. Fade away.

Coming out of the trance

And now I'am going to count from one to five and I will say, your eyes are open, you are fully aware, feeling refreshed, relaxed, renewed, totally, totally at peace with yourself and with the world around you. Enjoying a sharp mind, a clear head and a tranquil heart. One – slowly, calmly, easy, gently, beginning to return to full awareness once again (clear throat), enjoying a sharp mind, a clear head and a tranquil heart.
Two – each muscle and nerve in your body is loose, limp, relaxed and you feel wonderfully good. You feel at peace with yourself and with the world around you. Enjoying a sharp mind, a clear head and a tranquil heart.
Three – from head to toe, you are feeling so much better in every way. Physically better, mentally better, emotionally, cool, calm and serene. Enjoying a sharp mind, a clear head and a tranquil heart.
Four – your eyes begin to feel sparkling clear as if bathed in cool spring water. And now Five – eyelids open. Open your eyes. Fully aware.

Suzanne: Ahhh hahhh hahhh.

Anny: Take a slow deep breath. Fill up your lungs and give yourself a pretty good stretch.

Suzanne: (stretch) Ummm. Well that was interesting.

Anny: What surprised you??

Suzanne: Yah, yah I thought I knew where it came from and it did not. Yahh, it went way, way back further than I ever imagined.

Anny: How does it feel here? *(Indicating where the feeling was in her body)*

Suzanne: Fine.

Anny: You like that?

Suzanne: Yah, yah, yah it feels good.

Anny: Your mind goes there and I thought you would love it like that and you wanted to stay that way. Anything else?

Suzanne: How vivid it was. It really surprised – well it did surprise me. Like the blue was so electric. It was just. I did not know they wore that kind of stuff, but just electric in that it had all these pointy little. Like the skirt. And gold on it with the blue and dark features, dark hair. Yah, it was just dark skin.

Anny: Okay.

Suzanne: It was quite surprise. And the tomb was very real.

Anny: Umm humm.

Suzanne: And now I understand that why when the door shut at night is when I felt it. It is the dark and when the door shut, it was like the closing off.

Anny: So, how is it going to be for now?

Suzanne: Okay.

Anny: All right.

Suzanne: Yah, I think, I know, okay. I stood in

Anny: Okay.

Suzanne: In our bedroom and it felt okay. It felt like the universe to me. Not like a ..

Anny: Okay.

Suzanne: Yah.

Anny: Very good.

Suzanne: Yah, it felt better. Much better. So that was a past life? Like I don't..

Anny: I will tell you that tomorrow.

Suzanne: Okay because…

Anny: The thing is that all I am going to ask you to do, be careful with what you eat tonight.

Suzanne: Ohh, okay, meaning?

Anny: That because there is quite a shift of energy there.

Suzanne: Okay. There was a detached sense there when he was going over. It did not really feel like me, so, but yet, so I do not know. That is why I asked.

Anny: I will tell you tomorrow.

Suzanne: Okay, okay.

Anny: What I would like you to do is make sure that before you eat anything tonight. Just have a good look at it and then when you put it in your mouth, you will feel right away because there is quite a shift of energy there.

Suzanne: Ohh, okay, sure. Yah, I have questions because of that. Because I thought it was till we did other things and then it was different. Something that, I do not know. I do not know. Well maybe.

Anny: That is okay, what counts is that you feel great.

Suzanne: Ohh yah, I feel wonderful.

Anny: Okay.

Suzanne: Or if he was a part of me. I have got questions, yah, because it is like, it is different than I ever thought about it.

Anny: You are right. And remember what counts, is you are fine.

Suzanne: Yah, for sure.

Anny: That is all what counts. Okay.

Suzanne: Yes, thank you.

Anny: So I am going to stop those things and I will have my hug and then we will remove all those wires. They are for sound, right. Okay.

Questions About Aaron's Surrogate Session

- Question 1 -

- Question 2 -

- Question 3 -

- Question 4 -

- Question 5 -

Transcript – Aaron – Surrogate Session

A Letter From Aaron's Mother Requesting A Surrogate Session

Anny

Here is a list of some of Aaron's personality changes and behaviors that are harmful.

He get instant mad and violent very abusive. Physical, verbal/emotional, has stole money from me. I have observed that Aaron gets really mad he directs his anger towards females – Aaron uses his size to intimidate others.

He gets glossy eyed.

He has periods when his body odour is very bad. Sometimes it seems as if he has no hearing – when he looks at me it is as if there are another pair of eyes looking at me.

Lying.

Fear of bugs.

Thanks, Jane

Aaron's Surrogate Session

Anny: This is Anny Slegten, and we are Thursday, January 8th, 2004. This is a surrogate session. Healing at a distant session for Aaron at the request of Jane.

Lead the surrogate into a trance.

Facilitator: Okay, so I would like for you to please watch my fingers and as you watch my fingers and you listen to my voice, take a deep breath in, slowly exhale. Close your eyes.

And as you close your eyes, you feel yourself relaxing. Your muscles are relaxing, as your body is sinking deeply into the chair, your mind is becoming very calm and quiet.

And with the sound of my voice you feel yourself going deeper into relaxation. Into that wonderful state of hypnosis. You are relaxing completely your body and relaxing completely your mind.

Ask for protection and affirm the surrogate's space

And I am asking for your protection and well being and I say, God please allow only good things to come to us. And for this blessing, we give thanks. And now you ask to be put into the protection of your light. Your very own spark of light. It is at the centre of your chest. Allow that light to shine. Let it shine. Let it shine throughout every cell of your body. Throughout your aura, cleansing your body, cleansing your aura. Strengthening your body, strengthening your aura. And extending itself at one arm's length above you, beneath you, on each side of you, in front of you and behind you. And mentally repeat with me, this is my body. This is my space. Only light can come to me. Only light can come from me. This is my body and this is my space. Only my light is here.

Ask the surrogate to check the "security" of their own aura

And take a deep breath in. Slowly exhale. As you go deeper into relaxation I would like for you to look at yourself. Your body and your energy and make sure everything is intact and then let me know when it is.

Anny: It is, thank you.

Ask the surrogate to bring the client in front of them

Facilitator: And now ask Aaron to come to you and when he is here, let me know.

Begin the session

Anny: He is here all right. And it is like I am looking at Aaron and I am not looking at him really. You could almost say I am looking through him and I am asking to speak to the person who is outsmarting us. Because I know Aaron had a lot of different kind of therapy, direct and indirect. There is a part there that is outsmarting us and I want to connect with that person. I want to speak and connect with the person, whoever that is, that is outsmarting us. And there is something dark starting to come from behind. Starting to shape itself and it is coming – starting to show it from behind him.
Yah, good evening.

Facilitator: And as you are aware. Is this energy, does it have a name and could you describe it?

Anny: At the moment, it is like a pointed hat but it is dark. It is like a pointed hat that is starting – but not that wide – that is starting to show itself from behind Aaron. And I can sense a chuckle, although I do not see anything. Just a dark grey. Not black. It is not black. It is dark grey, and I can sense a chuckle, yah.
You are outsmarting us, don't you? Umm humm…
Absolutely…
And smells, humm…
Where did you get that smell?

Facilitator: What does it smell like? Is it....

Anny: Humm?

Facilitator: What does it smell like?

Anny: It smells, the odor of someone who has been very angry. Yah. Someone who has been very angry has a body odor and he has quite an odor that just came up.
However, he is chuckling...
So umm, yah.
Tell me, what is creating that smell? That very particular smell...
Okay. It is quite interesting:
What I see is energy more than a person because when I ask what is it that creates that smell, it is almost like a firework there. You know, it is just like a thing that has sparks coming out of a place where something electrical is about to start to burn.

Facilitator: Okay.

Anny: Yah, and really, it is quite amazing.
All right, so can you explain to me, what gets you in that mood?
Humm. I shocked him (laughter).
Okay. I would like you to remove your costume so I can see you.

Facilitator: (cough)

Anny: All right. He removed his costume really.
It was a costume and here I see... hahh...
A black man. He is black. Yah, he is black. Now how did you get black? Is it your colour or... Okay, it is someone who got burned. Umm humm. Because the way I looked at it. I am very familiar with black people and that was not a black person. Umm umm

Facilitator: And maybe that is why you saw the sparks. Like something before.

Anny: Umm humm. And there was smoke and sparks. The person was burned pretty bad, hey. He said yah, it was pretty bad. And let us go back there. I would like you to go back to before you got burned.

All right. Umm. I can see a young man. Umm. Well, is that interesting. He shows me that… Humm…

Here is what happened. He is showing me what happened. And it is that he was young, full of life and he was working. It has something to do with electricity. And it has something to do…

There is something about electricity there. Full of life, a young man and he was working at this industrial accident. He was working with… I am trying to figure out what does that have to do with electricity.

Well, I am going to get a lecture here… Ahh, he was a welder. It is not… yah it is electricity. It was, he was a welder and he is welding something that exploded. And he got really burned.

He was so black. He was so burned. And died from it. I am asking him what… Okay. Ohh. And he was, there was a co-worker with him and he says according to him, the co-worker… it is not a co-worker: It was a kind of a guy who was distributing the work giving that work, according to him, so that he would get killed and get out of the way.

Facilitator: Ohh.

Anny: Umm humm. Because I keep seeing a woman in this. And was he ever mad. When he got out of his body, he was so mad because he could see the set up. He realized the set up of the accident as he died. And he looked at the body. The body was all black.

Facilitator: And as he was looking at his body and realized the set up, what did he do after that and how is he feeling?

Anny: He decided he is going to get even with that guy and guess who is that guy? Aaron.

Facilitator: Umm. Okay.

Anny: Yup. He decided he is going to get even. And he is showing to me how he is messing up Aaron the way, at the time he messed him. Quite whooo!! Quite a vengeance there.

He said you better believe it. You are that angry? He said yup. He had a whole life in front of him and here it is, poof. Welding. It was an electric welding thing. It was in the beginning that it started to exist, so it is quite recent, while quite recent. 50 years ago, something like that.

And he said he knew it would explode because when he got out of his body and he saw the person who gave that job, he could tell crystal clear that that guy wanted him out of his way.

There was a competition for a girl. And is he ever mad. Is he ever mad. Ohh. And rightfully so. Umm humm… But then, is that giving you a life. You are stuck here. This kind of a vendetta type of a thing. So I can tell you, he was waiting. He said you better believe it, you just wait.

Facilitator: In read him, would you get to be the same age, or did he, or was it awhile for him to find Aaron there.

Anny: I did not get that.

Facilitator: Was he waiting for Aaron to be a certain age, or did it take him awhile to find Aaron?

Anny: Ohh no, he was looking for it. For him. He was. He said you wait, I will get even with you. And it was not a co-worker, it was the guy giving the work. He was much older than him huh.

Facilitator: Okay.

Anny: Yup, because Aaron at that time was much older than him and he was so mad because he had the whole life in front of him and he says to me.

It was obvious, it was jealously that made him do that. Because he was young his whole life and they both eyed the same girl and the guy was older. He was younger. And guess what, guess who got the favours. And he was so mad.

Ahh, was he mad. He said, you wait, get even with you. And he says that is Aaron. He is the guy. But then I am asking at what time did you attach yourself to Aaron? He said the time was right when he was 6. The time was right. And he decided he is going to ruin Aaron's life, the way he ruined his. Well, all right. I would like to address myself to you. How do you want me to call you? Rene comes up.

Facilitator: I'm sorry?

Anny: Rene.

Facilitator: Aaron?

Anny: No, Rene. R E N E.

Facilitator: Ohh, Rene. Okay.

Anny: Rene. It is Rene. I am asking him. Is it Rene?
He just looked at me with a weird look. He said that will do. Okay, so it is not Rene. I understood Rene. He said yes, it is Rod, Rodney. Ohh, okay, Rodney. Rodney, do you realize something, but first of all have a look at what is happening with Aaron for the last 10 years and how is it getting.

How it is getting.

He said yah, I am getting even all right. Look at his size. Okay. The temper, umm humm. The anger.
You are angry, right Rodney. He said yup. Well, do you realize that all this time you spent doing that, you do not have a life really.
Sure you are getting even, but then really you do not have your life.

Facilitator: You can have your own physical body and you could have many things.

Anny: You could have your own physical body, a beautiful life, a girl in your life, you could have, she could be a wife, you could have your own children, you could have your own shop maybe, I do not know.

Because obviously you remember being a welder don't you, so you could become quite a good welder by taking that knowledge back into the next life. You could even be your boss. The boss of a welding shop. Can you imagine? Umm humm.

Do you realize that your anger keeps you stuck. Umm humm. You like that thing, don't you.

The first thing I will ask you Rod, shed that burned flesh. Get back to your body the way it is supposed to be. Umm humm...

Do you not feel better now. Umm humm. Okay.

Now, I would like you to… Would you like to have your own life, first of all? Umm humm.

For that you will have to go through the light. You know that, do you? So, before you do through the light, how about taking all your stuff out of Aaron.

The whole thing. So that you leave him on his own really. With his own stuff. Umm humm.

So take the whole thing that belongs to you. The anger, everything that you are… that you have put into Aaron so that he is the way that he is: Lack of grooming, lacking of cleanliness, no honesty at all. Absolutely impossible to live with. Take it all out. And also the odour.

Take it all out. Because you know, as long as he has it, you are stuck. So you want to set yourself free, do you? So you have to take it out of there. Rod, take it out of there.

I will explain something. It is exactly the same. All those feelings are keeping you stuck, just like if you had given him a kidney or I do not know, an organ of yours. You will get stuck there.

Well guess what, all those feelings are keeping you stuck, because they are yours. So take it out of there. All right.

Facilitator: How is it going?

Anny: It is going quite well. The thing is that he – I m going to ask him now, he did not clean the head and I would like you to clean the head please.

Facilitator: Umm humm.

Anny: Take it all out. You want to set yourself free. Umm humm. Trust me on that Rodney. You better take it all out, everything that is your's.

Facilitator: He will be so happy when he knows that when he had all of that from the past to be burned and being transformed into something wonderful for him.

Anny: Umm humm.

Facilitator: The freeing the soul so you can have the next life free and enjoyable.

Anny: You know what, you are a welder don't you. Well, but then you have also… you can also use a torch to weld, don't you...
Yah, well you get it all out there. But do it safely this time, okay. Put the torch to it because it is your's and you want to get rid of it completely. Umm humm.

Facilitator: There is no feeling compared to feeling free.

Anny: Umm humm. Now, Rod, I am looking at you. You are good looking man. And you are going to go through the light aren't you. And I would like you to have something in mind there that the next time around, you will be healthy, good looking, handsome, wealthy, have a heart of gold, being highly intelligent and have a very wonderful life. I would like you to have that in mind. And go through the light. (deep breath) Now I am looking at Aaron.

Facilitator: And has Rodney gone into and through the light?

Anny: Oh, he went through the light. He just went. It is like, almost like there is a vacuum and he got, just like a fan will draw the smoke so to speak. Rodney went into kind of a vapour thing and got sucked in by the fan really. The exhaust fan type of a thing and he went. So now let's have a look at Aaron. Umm humm.

Facilitator: Where is Aaron's energy? Is his energy in his body at all, partially, or…how much of him was taken up by Rodney?

Anny: Ohh Rod was ohh ohh. Rod was taking a lot. I am asking Aaron to look at his light now and let it shine throughout your body, throughout your aura, flushing out whatever residue has to be flushed out. And at the same time, filling your whole body, your whole body with your very own energy. Umm humm.

Facilitator: And as he does, as that light is shining and he is updating all of his cells, muscles, nerves and bones in his body, he is also clearing his mind and correcting all the connections and they are flowing evenly, easily making up his mind, through his light in his body.

And I am asking your subconscious mind Aaron to heal, clear and resolve whatever should be healed and cleared and resolved. And once it has been healed, cleared and resolved, let me know in a gentle and easy manner.

And as this light of yours is shining through your body, there is also a shift and a change happening at deep level, the soul's level. You will notice the change in your behaviour and in your attitude and in the way your body feels as you are feeling your energy through every cell, every muscle, every nerve, every bone in your body.

Your body is feeling different and lighter, feeling very healthy and you notice as this shift and change is happening, your habits, your behaviours are shifting and changing as well and your body is becoming much more energetic and you are enjoying being at a weight that is healthy for you. For your height and your bone structure.

You are feeling your energy and as this energy flows through your body and is clearing the connections, in your mind, in that light of yours in your physical body, it feels wonderfully. This feeling is quite new and different, feeling your energy. How is it going?

Anny: It is going quite well. I see his aura now. He did not have one before.

Facilitator: Umm humm.

Anny: Now I see Aaron's aura.

Facilitator: And I am asking for your energy, Aaron, as you are aware of your light and it is flowing through your body and updating your cells and bones, muscles and nerves, all of that it is strengthening your body, healing your body and strengthening and healing your aura and your aura is becoming very strong with a protective cover so to speak around it. So that only your energy is in your body and your space. It is growing stronger starting now and into the future. Just strengthening and healing.

Anny: Now I am going to do something because he wants to leave, so I said allow me to put something in your heart so that you can have compassion, yet be firm, having self-respect as well as respect of others. And he is gone. He is gone.

Ask surrogate to say anything else they would like about the session

Facilitator: Do you have any comments?

Anny: The only comment I can say is that Rodney was quite angry. Very, very, very angry. Was he ever. It was real vendetta. And he did not realize that by doing that, he was cutting himself off of life. So that did it. The moment he realized that. Because he was going to go along and leave things in Aaron's head and when I saw that I said: you better clean it out too because remember whatever you leave that is your's, will keep you stuck.

He said all right. (laughter)
And when I asked him to get back into his healthy body, it was almost like all the black that was burned was just like… like it fell, it was like you would peel off a …

Facilitator: The paint of an oil painting?

Anny: Yah, but you know, yah when paint starts to flake, it was exactly that. And he just left – shooo. That is it.

Facilitator's Notes

Looking through Aaron – not Aaron himself.

Want to speak to the person who is outsmarting us.

Something dark came out from behind Aaron.

Seeing 'dark grey' can sense a chuckle.

Has a 'smell' – the odor of someone who has been very angry.

Sparking energy coming from him (like something electrical before it starts to burn).

Remove your costume – see a black man - black from a burn.

Go back to before you got burned.

See a young man full of life – working at welding – it exploded and he got burned and died.

There was a co-worker with him – he was set up to be killed by him – over a woman.

He is going to get him back – vengeance very strong.

He is very angry because he had his whole life ahead of him.

Rodney is the guy – what time did you attach yourself to Aaron?

Six years old.

René is his name – Aaron (?)

Look at the last 10 years with Aaron:
> His size
> Anger/temper

Rodney shed the burnt skin.

You could have your own life.

Take all your own stuff out of Aaron.

Go to the light – have something in mind – healthy, handsome, heart of gold, intelligent and have a wonderful life.

Looking at Aaron – Rodney had taken up a lot of his physical body.

Aaron's light to shine – strengthening and healing him in every way.

Putting something in Aaron's heart:

> Compassion and strength
> Self-respect and respect for others.

NOTE:

Jane, the one who asked for the session reported she knew immediately that we did the session: the body odor was gone!

Questions About Gary's Surrogate Session

- Question 1 -

- Question 2 -

- Question 3 -

- Question 4 -

- Question 5 -

Transcript – Gary – Surrogate Session

February 09, 2016

Anny: We are Tuesday, February 09, 2016. This is a surrogate session, a healing at a distance session for Gary at both his request and his wife's request. They are both agreeable to the idea. And the session is a healing session for everyone concerned so from what I, what it means is that it will benefit Gary and also everyone else around him. And it will benefit him at all levels. My name is Anny Slegten, clinical hypnotherapist and my facilitator is also a clinical hypnotherapist trained in this modality.

Facilitator: Okay, so are you ready?

Anny: Oh yes and I have that smiling face, you are looking at me.

Facilitator: As you take a slow deep breath and you exhale, you sleep now, sleep now. And you know when I say sleep now this is not the sleep that you fall asleep at night but that hypnotic sleep. Where you are relaxing your body and completely relaxing your mind, so your subconscious mind is open and very receptive to the suggestions you are receiving now. And as you go into this deep state of relaxation, you feel your body sinking deeper into the chair. Feeling more and more relaxed, calm and peaceful. And you become aware of your light, that spark of life in the centre of your chest. As it is shining throughout your body and out into your aura, you are feeling wonderfully good. Very bright and strong and your energy is contained in your body and your space. And I'd like for you to check our your energy, mine and the energy of this room to be sure it is all right and good for the work we are about to do.

Anny: Mine is very bright, so is yours. It is quite strong, the whole thing, the room, it is very synchronized so to speak, it is really very, very good, very clear, very everything.

Facilitator: So then you ask Gary to come to you in his own energy and when he is here let me know what you become aware of.

Anny: Oh he is here, and he has quite an inquisitive look to his face. You know he looks at me and said well what are you going to discover? I do not know, that is the reason we are doing this. Let us see, I would like you to stand in front of me. Hmm. You really wonder, don't you.

Okay, I am asking Gary to slowly turn. I want to see, I want to slowly turn so that I can see him from all sides. And I find it very interesting that it is something, you know, the root chakra there, it is that energy field really, because I do not know, the genitals, there is something there, but coming from the back of him. And it is only on a little bit, it is like, and it is from the back, I can see it from the back. I know it is behind him. And it is kind of a dark grey, and it is something that is looking and then hiding, looking and hiding.

What is happening with Gary? What's happening? And whatever it is, now it looks like it is straight behind him but whatever it is, is a little taller than Gary, Gary. Yeah. A little taller than him. So, huh. Whoever it is, whatever it is, can you put your, come on the side so I can see you? Yeah, just come on the side so I can see you. Hmm.

It is a man that was behind him. Something quite unusual. It is yeah, it is an entity, okay, behind him. Isn't that interesting, that really jealous of Gary, because of the type of wife he has. Hmm. That entity likes Gary's wife. So, he figures by attaching himself to Gary, he would have the advantage of Gary's wife. Hmm, isn't that something.

Facilitator: And what's happened?

Anny: She doesn't want anything to do with it. And he gets pretty mad. And wonders how come. How come is that although she cannot see it, he did not what we call "possess" Gary.

What he did and she cannot see it, make him, make him wear his clothes and everything so that he, in his imagination, is experiencing lovemaking of Gary with his wife.

Oh okay.

Anny: The thing is, he did not possess him. No, no. He just, he make, he make Gary, he in his mind Gary represents him.

Facilitator: Oh okay.

Anny: Okay? He is, yeah. He did not do that. And I ask him how come. It is because there is something about Gary that you don't go in.

Facilitator: Oh. That's good.

Anny: That's pretty good. The thing is, he really likes that wife. Ooh, she is hot, he says. I say how do you know that? He said, well he observed it and my God, he likes that type of lovemaking so that's how come he want it. Hmm. In French we would say, huh huh. He was, what we say in French, (Ce rinser l'oeil) that means he was baiting his eyes at her. It is, I don't know how do you say that in English, but in French, (Ce rinser l'oeil) , is a very precise thing. The thing is, what is interesting, he did not possess, he did not possess Gary. He made him look, in his idea, he make him look like, make Gary look like him so that it was easier for him to imagine him in bed with Gary's wife. The thing is that, he said, it doesn't work very well.

Facilitator: No, it would be better if you would go get your own body again.

Anny: The thing is that, the thing is that you see, you have to understand that I'm talking to whoever that is there, that you have to understand that when you do that, there's something more than just what we look like. There is an energy. There is a chemistry between Gary and his wife. And you don't have that chemistry so it goes flat, right? He says, you better believe it, he says . . . So what is it that, where did that happen and everything? You know what the entity said? Lay people would call it ghosts, but it is an earthbound spirit. He said, the way those two are together, he said, you can spot it. Especially in his field there, you know, where he's at, he could see it. It was as vibrant as vibrant can be, he said, when those two are together so it was easy to see them. Where did you see them?

You know what? I'm surprised by that. The earthbound spirit said that, what he does, he goes into restaurants of the hotels, in the little restaurants. And that is where he says the interaction with people is the most, visible. You can really see it. When they are eating, you can tell the chemistry between people, when they eat. There is something there, and then you follow them in bed of course, to see what's happening really. But the thing is, that is where you see it, the chemistry between the people as they eat. Well you know, whoever you are, thank you, I never thought about that and I didn't know that. Thank you for that information. He said well you're welcome. He said, he does that all the time. I said, Oh. And when you do that, how does it end up. He said, I don't know how come, he said, he said he doesn't know how come but he goes flat. That is because there is no chemistry. Just like you would go and eat at the table with those people, the chemistry would be gone. There is a chemistry there. So if you want that for you, you know what? You better have a good look at you, look at your life and everything, you know at everything and then go through the light so you can take on a body to be able to experience that.

Facilitator: Yes.

Anny: He said that's a lot of work. No, it is just a decision to make. But then I'm looking at Gary there, with what he's wearing. I want his name. Is it, in English, people would call him Mike. But he said, that's not the way we say it in Spanish.

So Mike. When did you start to do that, you know? He said, oh, he said, it is a lot of fun. With all those people from other countries, especially Canada, he said. He said to me, you can tell they are from Canada. I said how do you know that? It is cold and they are hot. They are always so warm, so warm, so warm.

So okay. I can see now, Gary and his wife on a beach, laying in the sand. You know, the beach, the sandy beach. He said the chemistry with those two is really making everybody envious, he said, Mike said. So. And isn't that interesting, Mike, that entity, what he said to me, that and then he started to manipulate the whole thing and it went worse because he could tell it was not working so it went worse, he said. So he tried to fix it, in Canada he said, and it doesn't work. It went flat. Oh.

Facilitator: So it sounds actually Mike, a lot of work what you're doing now.

Anny: What did you say?

Facilitator: It sounds like a lot of work what Mike is doing now.

Anny: Oh yeah, the thing is, there is something though so as he is looking at this and he doesn't look, he start to back off a little bit. But not that much. So, chemistry is starting again but it is not, it is not Gary that felt the difference in the chemistry, it is the wife that reacted to that. That's how come it went flat, he said. And I mean flat, he said. He is not happy. Mike is not happy. He could not understand how somebody so hot get so flat all of a sudden. He said, that doesn't make sense. Oh yes it does.

So Mike. Can you remove your clothes and your stuff. Can you remove them from Gary please? Mmhm. Can you remove it from Gary please? Well, he said, you know, because really, Gary dressed better than that. What he wears is better than that. That was his best.

Mike said, he plays with that comment. That's his best. Yeah, but the thing is, you know what is interesting? By putting his clothes on Gary, Gary still had that, Gary's chemistry feelings there with his wife, were stopped by the clothing. Because the cloth is not of the energy field of our physical thing, it is something different.

So what happened is that the cloth really, sent the energy of Mike. And Gary's wife wants nothing to do with it. Because it was not Gary.

Facilitator: Right. Absolutely.

Anny: You know Mike, in a way that is quite a compliment to Gary. And to his wife too. He is not happy because he said, my God, those two, he would have really like to have experienced that. Well I thought Mexican people were quite hot. That's what people think, he said, but no. Oh okay.

Facilitator: But if you . . .

Anny: And you know what he says? He says many times you almost have to make a prayer before the wife would _____.

Facilitator: Oh my goodness. You go into the light you can choose a body of any nationality, or anything, any kind of looks, whatever you want.

Anny: Mike, remove those clothes. Take it off, Mike, take it off Gary's body. You know what? He even had put his underwear, that whole thing so it is, okay. Gary, can you turn around please so that I don't see the front of you. Because now Gary is naked and I would like Gary to put back his clothes on. Yeah.

So then Gary is laughing, he said my, my, my, right. So now, Mike, hey. Yeah. Can you imagine, even the underwear? Mike said well you know, with the Canadians they are always cold, he thought they even needed a t-shirt. My, my, my. Okay now. Let's stop laughing there because this is not laughing matter.

So now, since Gary is naked, I'm going to ask Mike to let Gary have a shower to really cleanse his energy perfect. So that everything is gone and that whatever that was drained out, Mike collected and put it in a bucket or whatever and put the clothes there, hold them up, which is what you did, he just took the clothes and hold them up and say so that it is your stuff.

So now, Gary had a nice shower. It was almost, it was water and a lot of energy in it. It was a sparkling, sparkling water, almost energy that was liquid. So now, so now, he is drying himself up. And yeah. I really want him to turn his back on me so that he is putting his underwear and everything. And now he turns around and he looks at me, he's find it really funny the whole thing. The thing is, what happened was not funny at all. But the thing is, but yes, my God, who would think of something like that. I don't know, but you name it, I heard it. That is something new again. And Mike now is next to Gary with the bucket there and then, whatever was drained it belongs to him. And then the clothes.

Mike, how long have you been doing this? He said I don't know, there is no time here. You are right, there is not time. How about taking all your stuff and going through the light there. He said, all that stuff? Yes, it belongs to you. You take it all. And go through that light, to a new you. Go through the light to a new you.

And so Gary, become aware of your light, the spark of life that you have within you. And let it shine throughout your body, throughout your aura. Putting the energy, your very own vibrant energy back. Yeah. Very, very, vibrant energy. Put it back, put it back where it belongs. In your own, where in your body it belongs to. That's what I should have said. That's right Gary. Is everything okay? And enjoy.

Enjoy, your relationship with your wife, physically absolutely, mentally, emotionally, physically, or spiritually I should say. And everything else you want, by being in that relationship, in the relationship with her. Yeah. And notice how your energy is back intact, much to your surprise and delight. Yeah. Much to your surprise and delight.

And Mike? You are standing there with that pail and your clothes. Go to that light. Just go there. Just go there. And he is gone.

Facilitator: Okay. Is there anything else for the record?

Anny: You know what, that's the first time that I see an earthbound spirit, instead of get into or attached to the aura or whatever, couldn't do it because the energy of Gary was too strong. So for him, for the earthbound spirit, the solution was to put his own clothes on Gary. But the energy of Gary was too strong. Yeah. It is the first time that, you know I'm doing this for such a long time, that the first time that the entity decide well, I'm going to put the clothes on and see.

Facilitator: Okay.

Anny: It was quite a, that is the biggest surprise because he did not attach and did not possess. And wants the wife. And that's it then.

Questions About Angela's Surrogate Session

- Question 1 -

- Question 2 -

- Question 3 -

- Question 4 -

- Question 5 -

www.success-and-more.com

Transcript – Angela's Surrogate Session

Surrogate Session – Foetus Angela & Mother Darlene

Facilitator – Anny Slegten

Anny: Well, we are going to do a surrogate session, a healing at a distance session, for Darlene's Foetus, and the purpose of this session is to be a healing session, for everyone concerned.

Anny addressing the class:
Now, also what I want you to dc is to be sure you keep your thoughts to yourself, just observe this with blank, because this is all with telepathy, and it is like radio waves so please keep your thoughts to yourself.

Anny to Surrogate:

And you are ready, don't you? You are ready since last night, when I mentioned that.

Alright. So now, stare at my fingers, keep your gaze on my fingers and listen to my voice. Your eyelids are getting so heavy so that all that you want me to do, is bring my fingers down, so close your eyes.

And enjoy the relaxation. Enjoy that feeling that is so familiar to you. And allow a feeling of relaxaticn to flow, from the top of your head, to the tip of your toes. It is as though everything is slowing down, everything is slowing down. And let all your cares fade away, fade away, fade away, fade away.

As I am asking for your protection and your wellbeing, and I say God, please allow only good things to came to Marie and me, Anny the facilitator, and for this blessing, we give thanks. And now, you ask to be placed into the protection of your very own light. Your very own light, your spark of life, it is like a mini sun in your chest. Some people can see it, some people can feel it, some people simply know it is there.

That light of yours, that very beautiful light of yours, let it shine, let it shine. Let it shine throughout every cell of your body, throughout your aura, cleansing your body, cleansing your aura. Strengthening your body, strengthening your aura. Expanding itself at one arm's length above you, beneath you, at each side of you, in front of you, and behind you, and mentally repeat with me, "this is my body, this is my space, only light can come to me, only light can come from me, only my light can be here."

And as you take a slow, deep breath and exhale, check your aura, your energy field, to make absolutely sure it is appropriate for the type of work we are about to do.

Surrogate: (Nods yes)

Anny: Thank you, how about mine.

Surrogate: (Nods again)

Anny: Thank you, and now, as you take a slow, deep breath and exhale, call the energy of Darlene. Call her up.

Surrogate: I'm getting a-

Anny: What?

Surrogate: I'm getting a feeling of a strong, male presence between me and a small female presence.

Anny: Is that right?

Surrogate: Yes,

Anny: Alright. Take a deep breath, and as you exhale do whatever is required to be able to get in touch with whatever is going on here.

Surrogate: The larger male presence seems to be very stand-offish. That's not exactly the right word, but not affectionate to the female energy who seems to be subservient, as well as smaller, and seems to allow herself to be held in the background of the male, who seems, I get the feeling controlling her, and overshadowing her.
He got here before you put me into a trance, and was standing between us. Not overtly threatening, but not open to our interference.

Anny: All right. What is the concern of that male energy?

Surrogate: He seems to be concerned with being in control, and yet disregarding the emotions of the female.

Anny: Alright can you do something so that we can do some work here? Can you put him in a kind of a cocoon or something so that whatever he does, stays around him?

Surrogate: He seems to be ok with just turning and looking away. His back to us, his arms seem to be folded across his chest. And she seems to be prepared to come forward. She's now closer than he is.

Anny: Alright, can you do something to make sure that the energy of those 2 is separated for this work.

Surrogate: I am going to open a light above them, and I'm going to put them each in their own rays. He is unimpressed, but she seems to be responding. But I am confident that the light is like, they're each in their own capsule rays, and he can't escape.

Anny: Can you thank him for his cooperation.

Surrogate: He'll shake my hand. He sort of nods, like that. (sideways nod)

Anny: Alright, so now what's happening with the female? What's happening to her?

Surrogate: She's starting to stand up a little taller, she's um, allowing her own aura to stretch out a bit, she's looking around. And she's still not quite looking at me, she's avoiding my gaze. So I'm going to offer that we go for a little walk. And it's a nice kind of walk area, with pine trees and there's a fresh breeze in our face, and the sun is shining now. She's walking a little bit taller. And she waves her arm like she's referring to the area around us. And she's standing a bit taller now.
I now get the feeling of the pregnancy. She's not very forthcoming, she's just happy to walk. I'm going to let her lead. And I'm walking right behind her now. The trees are getting taller and thicker. She seems happier.

Anny: What does pregnancy mean to her? What does it mean to her, to be pregnant?

Surrogate: Like glowing, she's like glowing.

Anny: Glowing.

Surrogate: She's protecting the life inside of her.

Anny: Can you ask her, what is it that the flow in the cord goes from the baby to her, instead of from her to the baby. What is it that creates that?

Surrogate: The baby is rejecting her.

Anny: The baby is rejecting her. Take a deep breath, and as you exhale, connect with the Foetus. What is it that the Foetus, that baby, that life in her womb, is rejecting?

Surrogate: I see it like a blackness coming from the baby to the uterus wall. I get the feeling that if the choice was now, the baby would abort itself. I'm not getting anything about the other two.

Anny: That life within her, what is it that she is rejecting? It is a little girl, what is she rejecting? What is it about her mother that she is rejecting?

Surrogate: I get the feeling of someone turning their back. Someone dressed like a pioneer.

Anny: Pioneer?

Surrogate: With a gray dress with white designs on it, an apron, turning away. A little child sitting on the floor. Very young. Just wearing a diaper. She's cooking. I think she's at the stove. And now I'm getting the male presence at the door of the cabin.

Anny: What does that have to do with Darlene now, that girl is rejecting Darlene?

Surrogate: The little kid is holding onto anger from being rejected. It seems very deep for a little kid. It seems really strong for a little kid. I still have the male presence at the door but he doesn't seem to be going in. And the child doesn't seem to acknowledge that there's someone at the door, and the woman doesn't either. I'm getting the feeling that she's angry, she's banging the pots around as she's cooking. She's not angry at the baby, she's angry at the man.
But I don't think he's really there. I think that's his soul. I think he's dead. I think he's dead and he's standing in the doorway. The child blames the mother for his death.

Anny: The child is blaming the mother for what?

Surrogate: For the father's death.

Anny: For the father's death. Take a deep breath, and as you exhale, ask the little girl within Darlene, what does that have to do with her own mother now?

Surrogate: It's payback.

Anny: It is payback. Can you explain to the little girl, she already lost 2, don't you think it is enough payback?

Surrogate: I almost get the feeling that the one who's alive is not sorry to see the other 2 go.

Anny: OK

Surrogate: She's just consumed in her own rage.

Anny: Consumed in her own rage.

Surrogate: I get the feeling that she doesn't move very much, so she's not – cause most mothers like to feel the baby move, and it's another way of holding herself aloof.

Anny: What would it take for the Foetus to accept life from her mother? What will it take now?

Surrogate: I just moved the baby ahead and showed her, her mom completely devastated, and she's starting to feel like maybe she's gone too far. Like now that she can see her revenge, she doesn't want it. So I'm kind of making her watch, and I'm trying to make her connect with her mother, who's crying. It seems to be, seems to be she's feeling now like she wants to protect her mother from that. But now she's confused. Now she doesn't want that anymore.

Anny: Anything you can do so that the blood is flowing again, from the mother to her.

Surrogate: I'm making them the same age, and having her reach out to her mother, and she wants to. They're holding hands and they're hugging now. They're very close, they're very, very close there.

I'm bringing her back into the womb, and I'm making her listen to her mother's heartbeat. Let her feel the rhythm. Let her feel the breath. Let the vibrations of her mother go through her and the amniotic fluid. I'm getting her to reach for the wall of the uterus and just touch it, put her hands against it. They're so tiny, they're not-

I think she's starting to, almost like her whole body is nursing, I feel. And I'm wrapping her in a pink blanket and turning the blanket into the uterus. And she seems now more like a baby who's being cuddled, rather than who's existing in spite of things. I think she's ready to make it work. There's a very deep connection. And I'm feeling that the man is watching.

Anny: Make sure he stays away, for now.

Surrogate: He's staying away, but he's not, he's not, his attitude is changing like the baby's. And it's like he wants to be part of the family, he's reaching for them. I'm concerned about an attachment.

Anny: Mm-hmm. Mm-hmm.

Surrogate: Someone's here for him.

Anny: What?

Surrogate: Someone is here for him.

Anny: Is that right?

Surrogate: He wants to stay, but she's asking him to go.

Anny: Who is she?

Surrogate: Darlene.

Anny: OK

Surrogate: And I think the baby's letting him go. So I'm opening the light for him and turning it gold. He still won't go. It's better, it's better for the mother, it's better for the baby to be whole within themselves. And it's time for him to go.

Anny: What does he want to convey? What is the message he wants to give them?

Surrogate: He wants to stay there and protect them. He wants to fill the obligation of staying with them. But that's not going to happen. He'll get another chance. He can come back with them in another life.

Anny: Mm-hmm. Also, from going through the light, there are things that he will be able to do to help them, that he cannot where he is at right now.

Surrogate: He's gone. Now he's shining on them. But he's got things to do. He's gone. But the woman who took him,

Anny: What?

Surrogate: The person who took him is still shining on the mother and the baby. A grandparent, from some life, grandfather of the man.

Anny: How is the baby now?

Surrogate: Sleeping.

Anny: Alright, can you make sure the blood flows now, the way it should? The pulse in the cord.

Surrogate: I'm letting the baby get the rhythm.

Anny: Anything you can do, to get the baby to stay, for the full term, to be strong, healthy, happy and beautiful?

Surrogate: I'm letting the baby, the baby's higher self, wrap the baby, string by string in a silk cocoon. Not only to keep it healthy in itself, but to protect it from any chemicals that might be released by the deceased Foetuses. It's spinning and floating in the amniotic fluid.

Surrogate: I'm telling the baby to allow itself to be healthy, to allow itself to be growing. To allow itself to live.

Anny: And how about to allow herself to be born in a natural way. A pleasant experience. Being born, it is like.

Surrogate: In a wonderful, bonding way that will bring them back, back to a wonderful time that they shared before.

Anny: How about Darlene now?

Surrogate: She doesn't seem to be fully in herself, if I can put it that way, she's not fully animated. I get the feeling she's off to the side, about an inch.

Anny: Can you put her back into her body? What got her out of her body in the first place?

Surrogate: I'm, the first thing that comes to mind is the in vitro. Doctors.

Anny: OK

Surrogate: She felt odd, she was evasive. It felt like she was uncomfortable with it and was trying to push herself up out of the way.

Anny: All right. Just tell her that as a result she's getting one baby in her body, and it is ok to get back into her body.

Surrogate: I'm getting her to breathe the mountain air and each time she does, she seems to pull herself back in, like you expand when you breathe, and when she exhales she pulls herself back a little bit more.
Now she seems to be brighter.

Anny: Anything you can do so she stays there?

Surrogate: I am asking her what she needs to stay there. She has got unresolved feelings from that time as well. I went right back. She was a busy person, she had a lot of responsibilities. She did not do anything out of cruelty. She did the best she knew how. She gained and she lost in that life. But she has to let it go.

Anny: Make sure she knows, this is another life, another time.

Surrogate: She ca not drag that behind her. She got to cut the chains. We need to give her something to cut them with. Or, I need her to figure out what she would like to cut them with. She has got a rock. This is going to take a little while. But she has got a rhythm.
She did not cut the chain at her foot, there is about 2 links on it. She is still working on it. But she realizes what she has done by leaving 2 chain links on. She just about got it. Just about. Just about.

Anny: Anything you can do so that she is totally, totally at peace with it, and accept that baby?

Surrogate: She's sitting down and she's holding it in her hands, and she's looking at the baby, she's allowing herself to love that life, and it's just dissolving. She stays sitting down, now she's hugging her abdomen and it's different than before, it's different than the first time. Now she's sitting up against a tree and she's looking content.

Anny: And how is the child responding to it?

Surrogate: The baby's just accepting it, just loving it, just being in the moment.

Anny: Anything that you can do so that the two are accepting each other?

Surrogate: They've got their hands against each other.

Anny: OK. And with each breath that the mother does, the baby is feeling better and better. And with each heartbeat of the mother, the heart of the baby is getting stronger and stronger. Both benefitting from the experience of the miracle of life, really. Allowing each other to live fully. That's right. Anything else you can do for those two?

Surrogate: I'm just trying to get them into rhythm with each other, like the waves in the field when the wind blows, just get them in the rhythm with each other. I'll let them sit together and have some time. I feel like they're gone.

Anny: Now, I would like to have some clarification about that male energy there.

Surrogate: Mm-hmm.

Anny: I did not understand, is that the male energy that went through the light, or is it someone living now?

Surrogate: No he went through the light.

Anny: OK that's the one that went through the light. OK thank you. And how is Darlene feeling about all this now?

Surrogate: Relieved.

Anny: Relieved. So, Darlene breathe in that feeling, breathe in that feeling of relief. As something inside of you has shifted, and something inside the baby you carry has shifted too. So that you can enjoy living in a healthy way. Very healthy. Feeling great in every way. And now, ask Darlene, anything else we can do for her today?

Surrogate: I did a little, have a look at the future thing, imagine yourself there and you can be there with her, holding the baby and playing with her.

Anny: OK

Surrogate: She's playing.

Anny: And how is she feeling now?

Surrogate: They're having fun.
Alright. Yah I can see them in a rocking chair.

Anny: When they are gone let me know. Anything the baby wants to do?

Surrogate: The baby seems kind of tired.

Anny: Ya. I-

Surrogate: I'm not getting a good feeling from the father.

Anny: The father?

Surrogate: Ya.

Anny: Mm-hmm.

Surrogate: Ya, I'm getting a not bonding feeling, if you will.

Anny: What does he require for him to feel comfortable with that?

Surrogate: He needs them to reach out and pull him into them, because they're just so focused on each
other. He needs to be brought in. To look up, smile at him, and reach for him. He needs to hold the baby. And he needs to rock the baby. He's feeling very left out. But now I can see him with them. They look happy.
Anny: Anything else? Can you put them into the future, the three of them?

Surrogate: Ya, that's where I've got them. She's not quite a year old, ten months.
Anny: Alright.

Surrogate: Now he's in the rocking chair holding her. It looks good.

Anny: Alright, when they are gone, let me know.

Surrogate: (Nods-yes)

Anny: Alright, take a deep breath now and as you exhale, become aware of your light. Your light, your spark of life. And make sure it stayed intact, if it did not, repair it now.

Surrogate: (Nods)

Anny: How about mine?

Surrogate: (Nods)

Anny: Thank you. So now, as you take a slow, deep breath and exhale, just relax. And allow yourself to go deeper, and deeper, and deeper in a wonderful state of relaxation. And contemplate your life, and whatever you want to improve or dispose of, put it in a box, at your left hand side. And when it is done, please say so. Whatever it is.

Surrogate: Mm-hmm.

Anny: Alright now, the only thing I want to know is it something that you want to get rid of or something you want to improve?

Surrogate: Get rid of.

Anny: Get rid of?

Surrogate: Mm-hmm.

Anny: Alright. Since you are a farmer, how do you get rid of things?

Surrogate: You bury them.

Anny: You bury them. No, I knew you were going to say that, but it stays in the soil. So we are going to-

Surrogate: I'd rather send it to the sun-

Anny: You want to send it to the sun.

Surrogate: Release the energy for positive use.

Anny: OK and allow that, so you are sending it to the sun to be burned up, consumed and transformed, into very beneficial energy, for you and know that by the time you are leaving this office tonight, this afternoon, the whole thing will be transformed into something very positive for you, physically, emotionally, mentally, spiritually and financially. And for this blessing, we give thanks.

And now, I'm going to count from 1 to 5 and then I will say, your eyes are open, you are fully aware, feeling refreshed, relaxed, renewed, at peace with yourself and with the world around you, enjoying a sharp mind, a clear head and a tranquil heart.

One, slowly, calmly, easily, gently beginning to return to full awareness once again, enjoying a sharp mind, a clear head and a tranquil heart.

Two, each muscle and nerve in your body is loose, limp and relaxed, and you feel wonderfully good. You feel at peace with yourself and with the world around you. Enjoying a sharp mind, a clear head and a tranquil heart.

Three, from head to toe, you are feeling so much better in every way, physically, mentally, emotionally and spiritually.

Four, your eyes begin to feel sparkling clear, as if they were bathed in cool spring water.

And on five, eyelids open, open your eyes, yes I know you don't want to open them, but take a deep breath, fill up your lungs, give yourself a good stretch.

Surrogate: So you felt that guy here too?

Anny: What?

Surrogate: That guy that was here at the very beginning, you never felt that, or?

Anny: Yes I knew it was something like that, it was a physical sensation when there is an attachment. I thought hmm, I wonder who that is?

Session Follow Up

Darlene

Information received from her mother and father:

She was in the hospital on the day of the surrogate session, on complete bed rest and of course very upset. She was in the Royal Alex Hospital. That is where I went on the day of your special session for her.

Even by the next day (27th) she was calmer and because everything settled down she was discharged home on Sept 30 07. A nurse had to see her at home daily though to assess the surviving baby. She had to see the obstetrician and get U/Ss weekly so had to travel.

Despite this as you know Angela thrived and because of a high blood pressure one week before delivery was re-admitted where she went into labour and delivered on November 17 07.

A Caesarean section was needed because despite rapid dilatation of the cervix and excellent pushing (which did push Angela about halfway through the birth canal), the angle of exit was altered – the twin remains and was partially obstructing the tract, and causing the head to push into the fairly narrow front bony pelvis . Also a section would have been needed to retrieve the twins.

Angela was born 6 weeks early (34 weeks) The twins survived until 27 weeks. Angela's birth weight was 4lbs.9ozs and she was very alert when born needing only to be tube fed due to immaturity for the sucking reflex.

Thank-You again Anny for the help.

One triplet died on Saturday, September 23 (27 weeks gestation)

The second triplet died the next day, Sunday, September 24

27 weeks gestation)

Awareness of the situation Tuesday, September 25.
(27 weeks gestation)

Surrogate Wednesday, September 26

Angela was delivered November 17, 2007 (34 weeks)

Accessing And Understanding A World Alive And Well

The Practice Of Surrogate Sessions – The Things Our Physical Eyes Usually Do Not See

The incredible beauty of going into a hypnotic trance is the discovery of who we are as human beings. It is also about discovering how we use the power of the Spirit within us to manipulate our inner power to our liking.

Thought Forms

A thought form is exactly that: The Energy we put in a thought takes form and becomes an entity, a person. It is the way curses are formed – usually during a particular ritual inserting Energy as well as a clear intent.

During a surrogate session – investigating something unusual – you can then obverse the complete scenario. It is fascinating to watch! It may also hone your skills at how to manipulate Energy.

There are as many ways to handle curses as there are people dwelling into this form of activities.

As you are reading this, please write down your questions on how to handle curses and Thought Forms. It will allow me to give you the information in a way you will then comprehend.

After all these years… I must admit I am getting good at this too – using it efficiently when psychically attacked. This is when my assertiveness comes into play and I am ruthless when defending myself.

Remember, being a Holistic practitioner does not mean we are Holy.

In HYP 101, I explained the subconscious mind is the switchboard between the conscious mind (the brain) and the higher self (our Spirit).

When regularly connecting with your subconscious mind, requesting clarity in a situation, your subconscious mind becomes a Thought Form. This is the reason I suggested you give you subconscious a name.

In my view, this is the highest source of information given to us as human beings. The subconscious mind opens the door to the vast pool of information in the Universal Energy Field.

When not having an answer, Subby (as I call mine) advises me I must rephrase my question.

Subby also advises me when a situation is about to happen. Sometimes with an overwhelming inner voice, a strong intuition, or through a clairvoyant dream. This always comes at the right time.

As you are reading this, please remember – there is nothing special about it. We all come from the same source. We all have the ability to experience both a clear head and an inner voice.

You have within you a Spirit (your Soul) that decided to have a physical experience. Therefore, allow your Soul to both experience living a physical life, as well as expressing itself as an inner voice or in a clairvoyant dream.

Who Are Discarnate Entities – Usually Called Ghosts?

As the body has released the Soul, the Soul finds itself without a physical body at what is usually called the planning stage.

Depending how a person dies **AND** they have been knocked out in the following ways:

- An accident
- In a coma
- Anaesthetized
- Heavily drugged
- Or intoxicated to the point of not be consciously aware of anything

The person is not aware of having left their body.

In these situations, the release of the Soul is usually smooth – leaving the Entity disoriented and wondering what happened to their body – or they are not aware they no longer have a body. They go on with their regular routine. This is regarded as 'a lost soul.'

Depending on their beliefs about the afterlife, and when they become aware they are at the end of their physical life – the way they perceive themselves is as varied as when physically alive.

The planning stage, sometimes called purgatory, is the time when an Entity takes stock of what happened during the life they just left. It takes courage for them to stay in purgatory, judging themselves, as they discover the only thing they took along is their consciousness.

Yes, we are the ones who judge ourselves – and we all know how we think of ourselves when we discover having done something wrong!

Having the courage to take a good look at themselves, they realize the best way to atone (according to them) is to undo their wrongdoing.

They do this with the intent of putting closure to what is sitting heavily on their conscious as they released their Soul.

It is at this moment that they write the script of their next life –

Others, in a hurry to go through the Light, bypass the planning stage. They do this in the hope to escape what sits heavily in their conscious, and find themselves repeating the life experience they just left.

They wonder how come life keeps repeating itself – life, after life, after life, after life – each time wearing a different coat.

Yes, we are the ones who make it this way. And however how hard it is to admit it, there are no victims, only volunteers.

When a session like this occurs, be aware: Both the attached Entity(s) as well as the person having reviewed a traumatic past life needs aftercare.

The Host specifically needs aftercare from having had an Earthbound Entity removed from their Energy Field.

Explaining the "what for" along with instructions for these sessions will be given during classes, with examples of what I have observed as well as what my clients taught me.

www.success-and-more.com

Afterword

As you are reading, and then studying the transcripts of various sessions, my intent is for you to be at peace. You are doing so as well understanding the benefits of being able to do surrogate sessions.

Sometimes an issue is derived from a learned behaviour. As you realize this – you will understand the issue is a decision frozen in present time. This is also known as mental block, a past life, or an entity attachment.

When going from effect back to cause, the issues are sometimes uncovered and resolved during a one-on-one session, or sometimes during a surrogate session. And sometimes, the only way to get a clear and precise understanding is by surrogate session.

I welcome your questions about this during class as I can give you many examples of one-on-one and surrogate sessions.

Observing the experiences of a soul when in physical form is fascinating.

We are truly one of a kind.

Going from effect back to cause – we discover we planned our own physical journey (details and all), during what is usually called the planning stage.

That we like it or not – discovering the reality of our "what for" allows us to realise we are the only one who has volunteered for our physical journey.

And, much to my chagrin… I am not exempt neither!

The result? An incredible understanding of our life experience and the inner peace that comes with it.

Anny

www.success-and-more.com

www.success-and-more.com

www.success-and-more.com

www.success-and-more.com

www.success-and-more.com

www.success-and-more.com

www.success-and-more.com

www.success-and-more.com

www.success-and-more.com

www.success-and-more.com

www.success-and-more.com

www.success-and-more.com

www.success-and-more.com

www.success-and-more.com

www.success-and-more.com

www.success-and-more.com

www.success-and-more.com

www.success-and-more.com

www.success-and-more.com

www.success-and-more.com

www.success-and-more.com

www.success-and-more.com

www.success-and-more.com

Online Store, Contact, And More…

You may contact Anny by visiting any of her websites and scroll down the home page to the contact information.

http://www.annyslegten.com
Anny's private website and online store.

http://www.success-and-more.com
To find the description of the many services offered, and more.

http://www.htialberta.com
The Hypnotism Training Institute of Alberta including descriptions of hypnosis and hypnotherapy courses given.

http://www.reiki-canada.com
About the Reiki Training Centre of Canada.

http://www.slegtenianhypnosis.com
Although open to anyone interested in this fascinating hypnosis modality, this website information is for graduates of the Hypnotism Training Institute of Alberta.

http://www.connectwithanny.com
This is the best place to keep up to date with Anny – including seeing all her latest books and how to order them on Amazon.

Other Books By Anny Slegten…

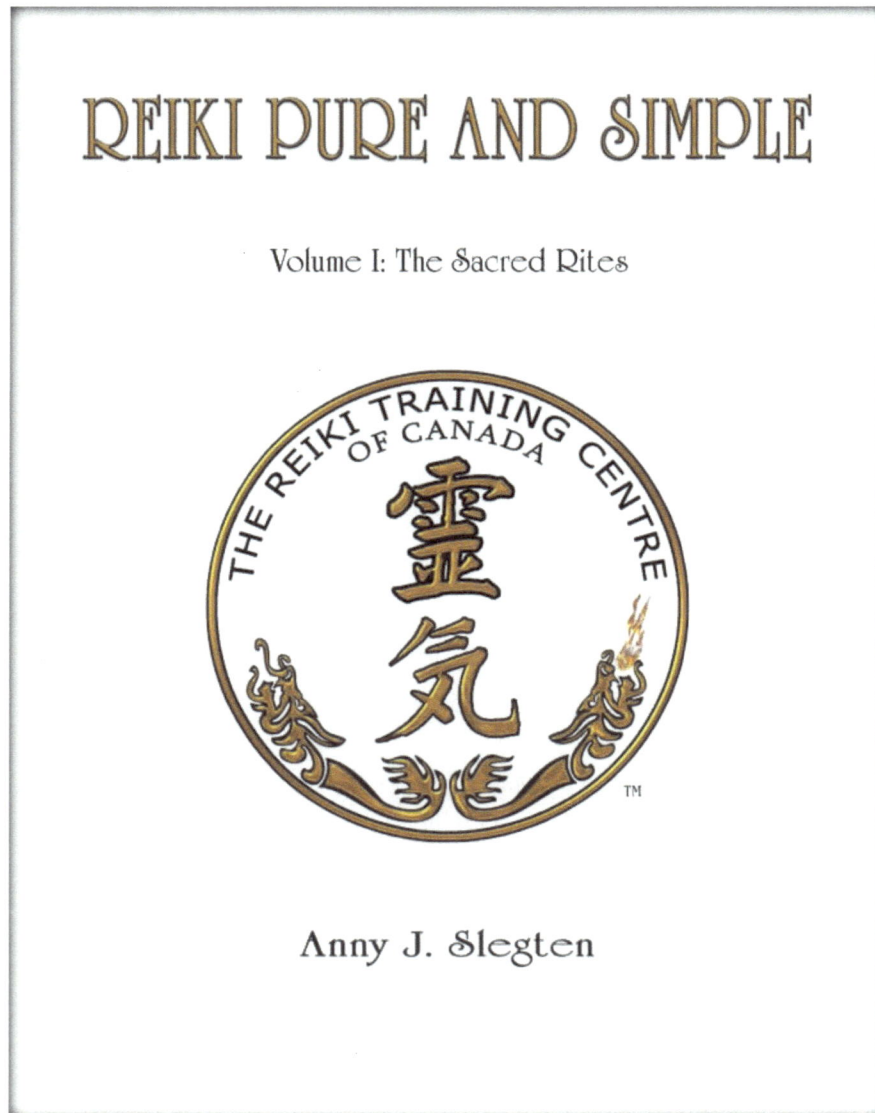

REIKI PURE AND SIMPLE

Volume I: The Sacred Rites

Anny J. Slegten

Reiki Training Centre of Canada
Class Material
http://www.reiki-canada.com

REIKI PURE AND SIMPLE

Volume II: Reiki Ryoho Hikkei
(The Most Important Methods for Reiki)

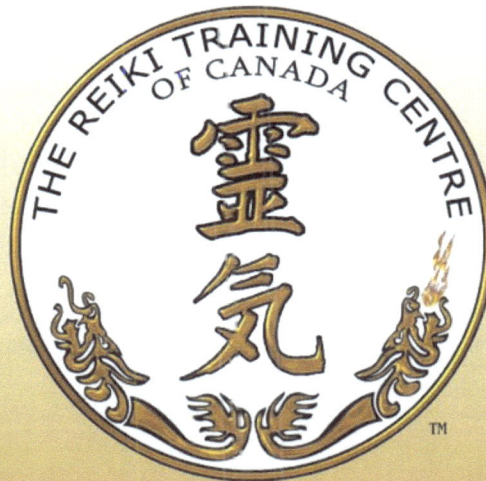

THE REIKI TRAINING CENTRE
OF CANADA

靈氣

靈気療法必携

Anny J. Slegten

This book is a must read for Reiki Practitioners
regardless of their spiritual lineage
and could be of great benefit to Energy Healers
http://www.reiki-canada.com

REIKI PURE AND SIMPLE

Volume III: The Many Ways of Reiki

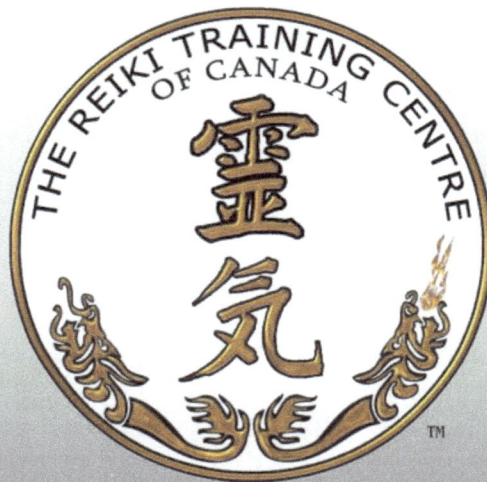

THE REIKI TRAINING CENTRE OF CANADA

霊
気

Anny J. Slegten

The Many Ways of Reiki
http://www.reiki-canada.com

REIKI PURE AND SIMPLE

TRADITIONAL JAPANESE REIKI

Volume IV: The Teacher Manual

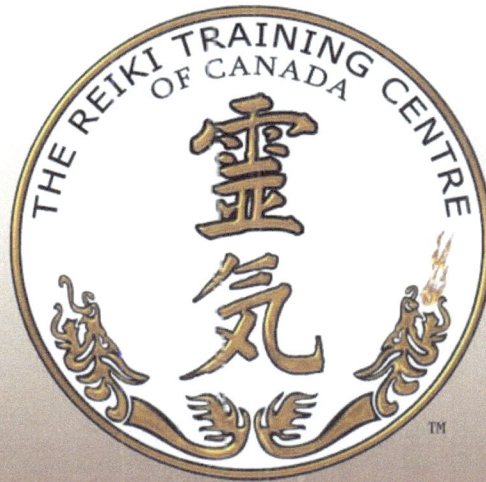

THE REIKI TRAINING CENTRE
OF CANADA

靈
氣

™

Anny J. Slegten

The Reiki Training Centre of Canada
Teacher's Manual
http://www.reiki-canada.com

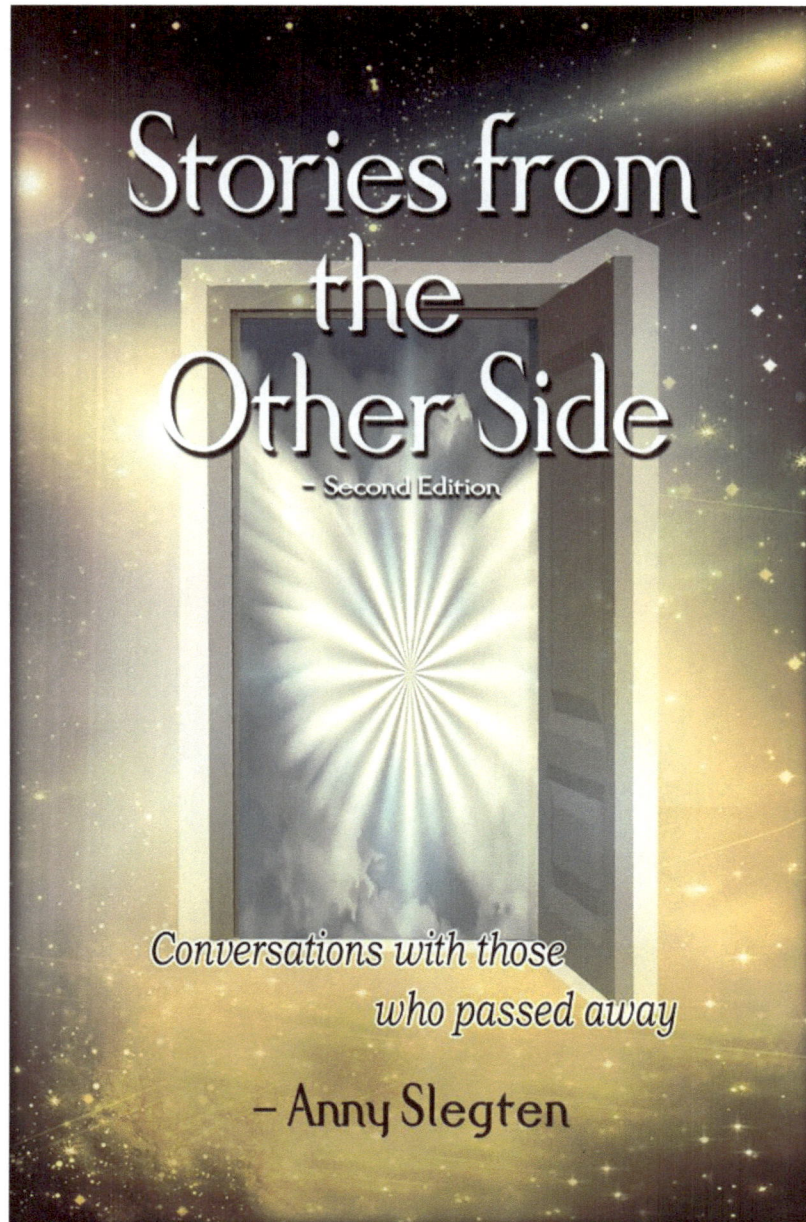

Stories from The Other Side – Second Edition
http://www.connectwithanny.com

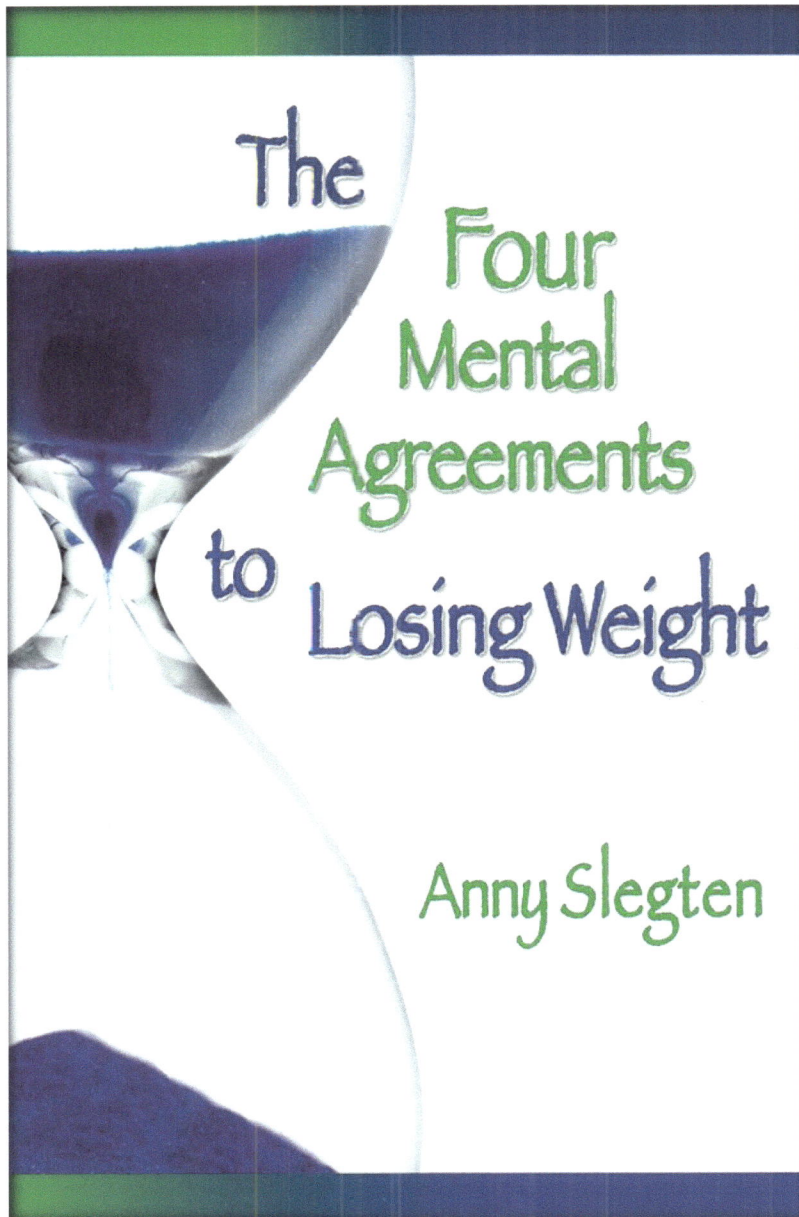

The Four Mental Agreements to Losing Weight

Anny Slegten

The Four Mental Agreements
To Losing Weight
http://www.connectwithanny.com

www.success-and-more.com

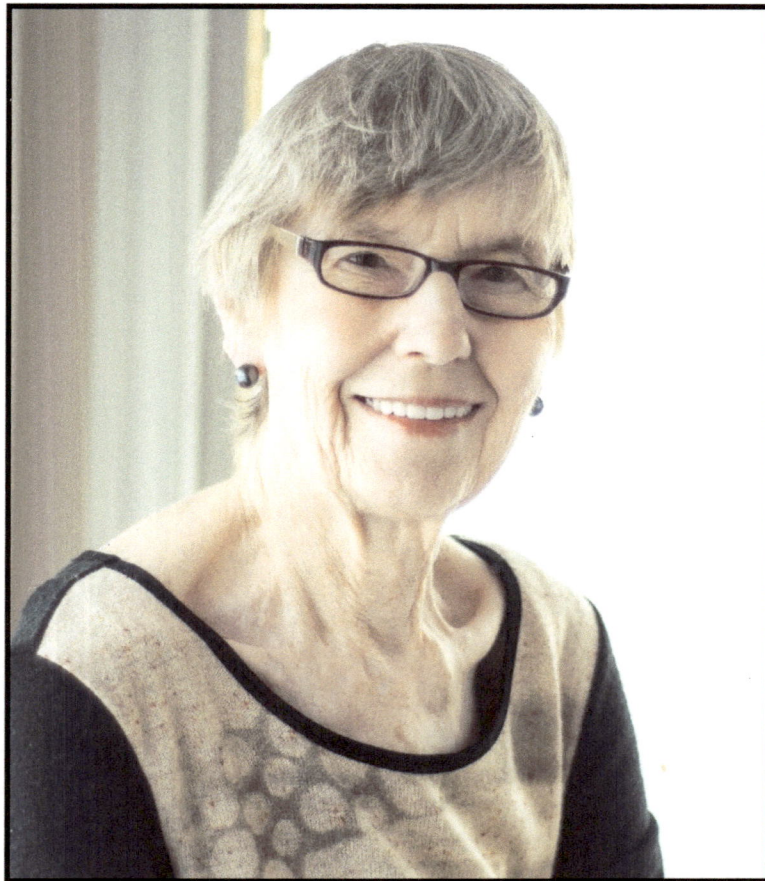

About The Author

As Director of The Hypnotism Training Institute of Alberta and The Reiki Training Centre of Canada, Anny has developed and structured the training and curriculum to the highest standards for both The Hypnotism Training Institute of Alberta and the Reiki Training Centre of Canada.

She offers training to students that come from all over Canada and around the world.

Anny has experienced and lived in many corners of the globe and this has given her a unique understanding of many cultures.

Anny's Belgian parents were from the Flemish part of Belgium and were

www.success-and-more.com

speaking Flemish (Dutch) at home. Living in Congo, everything was in French.

Although she never spoke Flemish (Dutch), Anny speaks English with a guttural Dutch/German accent. Living in the English-speaking part of Canada for decades, Anny now speaks French with an English accent!

Anny is an Author and holds certifications as:

Master Hypnotist
Clinical Hypnotherapist
Hypno-Baby Birthing Facilitator and Instructor
HypnoBirthing TM Fertility Therapist for Men & Women
Reiki Master/Teacher
Master Remote Viewer

Anny is a world renowned Clinical Hypnotherapist and Hypnologist in full time practice since 1984 as well as a Hypno-Energy worker since 2008.

In 1986 Anny created and developed an unique method using hypnosis for distance services - Virtual Sessions.

Over the years these Virtual Sessions proved to be an effective, useful, and efficient method for investigations and putting closure on both present and past issues - resulting in peace of mind.

To know more about Anny, please visit www.annyslegten.com and make sure to read what she published on her Blog.

Do you wonder what else Anny is publishing?

Visit www.connectwithanny.com

www.success-and-more.com

www.ingramcontent.com/pod-product-compliance
Lightning Source LLC
Chambersburg PA
CBHW050813220326
41598CB00006B/201